THE **CRUNCH** FITNESS GUIDES

GET FIT
IN A CRUNCH

CRUNCH

HATHERLEIGH
NEW YORK

GetFitNow.com Books
An Independent Imprint of Hatherleigh Press

GetFitNow.com Books
An Independent Imprint of Hatherleigh Press
an affiliate of W.W. Norton & Company
500 Fifth Avenue
New York, NY 10110
1-800-367-2550
www.getfitnow.com

Before beginning any strenuous exercise program consult your physician. The author and publisher of this book and workout disclaim any liability, personal or professional, resulting from the misapplication of any of the training procedures described in this publication.

All GetFitNow.com books are available for bulk purchase, special promotions, and premiums. For more information, please contact the manager of our Special Sales department at 1-800-367-2550.

Library of Congress Cataloging in-Publication Data

Crunch Fitness,
    Get fit in a crunch / Crunch.
        p.   cm.   —   (The Crunch Fitness Series)
    ISBN 1-57826-026-4 (alk. paper)
    1. Exercise.   2. Physical fitness.   3. Nutrition.   I. Crunch   II. Series.
RA781.G45   1999
613.7—dc21
                                                                99-34885
                                                                CIP

Series Editor: Heather Ogilvie
Cover design: Lisa Fyfe
Text design and composition: John Reinhardt Book Design
Photographs: Peter Field Peck with Canon® cameras and lenses on Fuji® print and slide film

Printed in Canada on acid-free paper

10 9 8 7 6 5 4 3 2 1

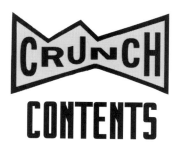

CONTENTS

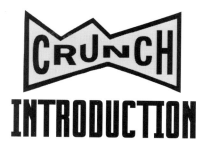

INTRODUCTION

Welcome to CRUNCH! For over a decade, we've been welcoming people of all shapes, sizes, ages, and fitness levels to our gyms. As we've expanded from a tiny, one-room aerobics studio in New York's East Village to cities across the country (and even to Tokyo), we've offered group fitness classes, personal training, and equipment to appeal to everyone from stressed-out workaholics and jet setters to senior citizens and expectant moms. We're living up to our motto, "No Judgements!"

We're aware that some people shy away from joining a gym or from starting a fitness program because they think it demands too great a change in their lifestyle. But at CRUNCH, we believe you shouldn't have to change your lifestyle in order to be fit. In fact, we believe your workout should change to fit your lifestyle. It is our firm belief that the success of a fitness program has nothing to do with how many hours you spend in the gym, but how good you feel when you're outside the gym, living your life.

That's why we've created these fitness guides—to show you that no matter what your lifestyle, there's a workout you can do that will complement it and get you fit. For example, we designed the *Road Warrior Workout* for people who spend a lot of time traveling on business. These folks don't have to give up their fitness programs—in fact, by doing a workout specially adapted to life on the road, they can maintain their fitness level and become less susceptible to all the common aches and discomforts of travel.

Get Fit in a CRUNCH is for those people who are trying to shape up in time for a big event—a wedding, a reunion, a trip to the beach. Based on CRUNCH's popular class, Emergency Beach Training, *Get Fit in a CRUNCH* lays out a safe, effective four-week workout, 12-week workout, and six-month workout.

Since the hardest part of any fitness program is starting it, we've written *Beginner's Luck* to help people stay motivated and become more familiar with—and less intimidated by—basic cardiovascular and strength training exercises. It's a workout you can take at your own pace, according to your own goals.

Look for additions to the CRUNCH Fitness Guides targeting time-pressed workaholics, first-time marathon runners, and people who want to eliminate or avoid common back pain and improve posture.

At CRUNCH, we don't want you to conform to some workout fad or a lifestyle of spending more time at the gym than at play. We want to give you workout options that will conform to your lifestyle—without judgement.

Doug Levine
Founder and CEO
Crunch Fitness International, Inc.
www.crunch.com

CRUNCH
ABOUT THE AUTHORS

Jonathan Watt, a trainer in CRUNCH's Los Angeles gym, designed the workouts in this book. Accredited by the American Council on Exercise, Jon is a post-injury rehab specialist, a stretch specialist, and certified in kickboxing to boot. He has ten years' experience in wrestling—and helping people who are wrestling with their weight and fitness. He's a firm believer in circuit training—switching back and forth among muscles groups during a workout to keep the heart rate up and burn fat while toning muscles.

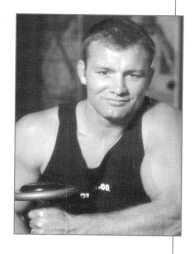

Brian Delmonico designed the stretching routine for *Get Fit in a CRUNCH*. A trainer in CRUNCH's 13th Street gym in New York City, Brian began his career as a gymnast at age 6. In his teens, he was on the National Gymnastics Team for three years, and he's a three-time All-American and two-time Big Ten Champion. He graduated from Ohio State University with a Bachelor's Degree in Education and Nutrition. Brian is certified by the USGF in Safety and Stretching—and he has a black belt in Tae Kwon Do.

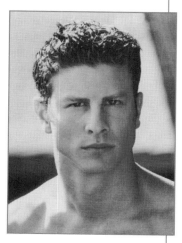

Larry Krug and **Jennifer Nardini** designed the nutritional program in Chapter 5.

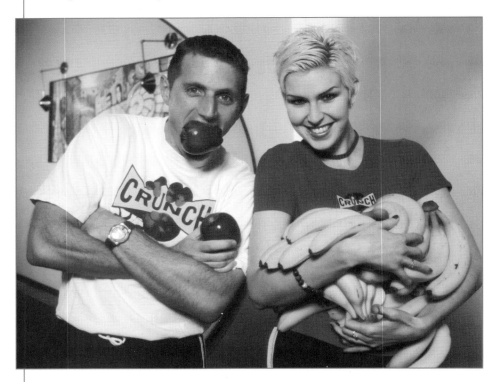

Larry Krug is the co-founder of the Eatwize™ Program. He has a Master's Degree in exercise physiology and served as a nutrition and training consultant for the 1996 Olympic Games. He has appeared on CNN, Dateline NBC, and E-Channel, and his nutritional and training advice has been covered in *Newsweek*, *Allure*, *Redbook*, *Cosmopolitan*, and *US* magazines.

Jennifer Nardini is both a professional journalist and personal nutritionist at CRUNCH Los Angeles. She is currently Head of Research and Development for the Eatwize™ Program and uses the method to help her own clients reach their goals. After graduating from the University of Washington with an education in both nutrition and journalism, she co-founded the Healthy Eating Rules (H.E.R.) Club, a nutritional and weight-loss support forum on the *Self Magazine* Web site. The H.E.R. Club can be accessed online at www.phys.com.

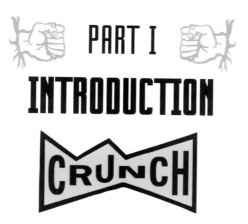

PART I
INTRODUCTION

Think it's too late to get in shape for a trip to the beach or a special event? Think again. If you're in a crunch for time, it's time for CRUNCH!

If you need to get in shape in four weeks, 12 weeks, or six months, you can rely on these comprehensive fitness and nutrition programs CRUNCH has designed for folks motivated by a fast-approaching deadline.

Easy to follow and effective, the GET FIT IN A CRUNCH fitness programs get your body in shape by increasing your metabolic rate: Each workout combines a healthy diet with cardiovascular workouts and strength training. CRUNCH nutritionists will give you the skinny on proper nutrition, you'll get top secrets from CRUNCH personal trainers, and the workouts will even target the body's "problem areas."

Bear this mind: These workouts are not just another set of "quick fixes" that might leave you looking good but feeling lousy. Our trainers have taken care to design programs that will help you look fantastic and feel fantastic! Your overall well-being is CRUNCH's goal.

Whether you want to get fit in one month, three months, or six months, we'll show you how to reach your fitness potential in the time you have. A single training philosophy underlies each of the workouts, so as you progress through the weeks, you'll understand—as well as feel—how the workouts are making you leaner and stronger. If you choose to do the Four-Week Workout, you'll probably want to continue a workout program when the month is up—and because the 12-Week and Six-Month Workouts are designed on the same principles, they'll be easy to pick up.

So what's your motivation? Is it your high school reunion next month? Is it your wedding in six months? Or is beach season right around the corner? Mark your calendar. Choose your workout. Now it's time to start the warm up—and the countdown.

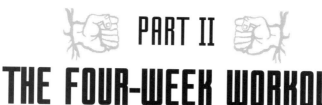

PART II
THE FOUR-WEEK WORKOUT

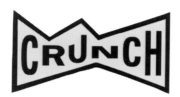

The Four-Week Workout is designed to shape you up in a month by increasing your metabolic rate. Based on CRUNCH's popular program, Emergency Beach Training, the Four-Week Workout combines a healthy diet with cardiovascular and strength training exercises. The first week consists of six workouts (three days of cardiovascular activity and three days of free weights) that will ready your body for the more rigorous weeks of activity that follow. Over the next few weeks you will raise the intensity level of each workout, thereby increasing your caloric expenditure.

However, in order for the Four-Week Workout to work effectively, you have to make a time commitment: CRUNCH personal trainer Jonathan Watt recommends setting aside one hour, six days each week—three for cardiovascular training, three for strength training— over the four-week program.

If you're doing the Four-Week Workout at home, we recommend purchasing the following exercise accessories:

- Hand-held dumbbells: 5 lb., 8 lb., and 10 lb.
- Jump rope

Remember, we're trying to shake up the system! So we've divided the cardiovascular workouts into two goals: fat-burning cardiovascular activity and an interval training cardio workout designed to increase your aerobic capacity. The Four-Week Workout includes three days of cardiovascular training each week, alternating the type of cardio workout each time. Your first week concentrates on intermediate, low intensity training aimed at reducing body fat and preparing your body for the more rigorous training that follows.

FAT-BURNING CARDIOVASCULAR WORKOUTS

These workouts consist of 30-minute segments of cardiovascular activity (walking, biking, rowing, etc.) of moderate intensity in your target fat-burning zone. The activity may be walking, jogging, biking, swimming, or any continuous activity in which you can maintain a specific intensity. The goal of this training method — known as slow distance training—is to sustain activity at 60 to 75% of your maximum heart rate.

Your maximum heart rate is determined by subtracting your age from 220. Let's use a 20-year old as an example:

220 minus 20 years = 200 beats per minute (bpm)

200 bpm = maximum heart rate

60 to 75% intensity = 120 to 150 beats per minute

Heart rate monitors offer the most convenient readings, but a more practical approach is a six-second pulse count. Count the number of beats felt in six seconds and multiply that by 10. For example, if our 20-year old counts 14 beats in six seconds, she is exercising at 140 beats per minute — well within her fat-burning zone.

STRENGTH TRAINING

The strength training element of the Four-Week Workout is based on the philosophy of interval training — keeping the body moving by continually alternating the exercises for each muscle group. By constantly switching muscle groups, you're making the heart work harder, thereby elevating the metabolic rate.

This workout uses dumbbells and jump ropes to put the body through a rigorous, one-hour full-body workout. Any medium-sized living room can serve as your exercise area. Be sure to allow 45 to 60 minutes for the workout.

The program is broken down into intervals of warm-ups/cooldowns, lower and upper body training, and two stages dedicated to abdominal conditioning.

20 aug ⟨1⟩

WEEK 1

DAY 1

Start off with 20 minutes of light, aerobic cardiovascular activity. The goal is not to overexert yourself the first day, but to identify your target heart zone. Find an activity you enjoy—biking, swimming, jogging, brisk walking, etc. Load up the Walkman and spend some time getting the blood and oxygen pumping through your body.

DAY 2

Here is a table of the exercises you'll be doing, followed by detailed descriptions:

Exercise	Reps / Time / Weight	
Warm up/Stretch		
Jump rope	60 seconds	
Break	60 seconds	
Jump rope	60 seconds	
Body squats	1 set of 15	
Knee push-ups	1 set of 15	
Step-ups	1 set of 15 per leg	
Bent-over, seated rear deltoid raises	1 set of 15	5 lbs.
Break	30 seconds	
Stationary lunges	1 set of 15 per leg	
Overhead shoulder presses	1 set of 15	
Plié squats	1 set of 15	
Bench tricep dips	1 set of 12	
Side steps	1 set of 20 per leg	
Dumbbell curls	1 set of 15	5–8 lbs.
Abdominal clams	2 sets of 10–25	
Jump rope	60 seconds	
Break	60 seconds	
Jump rope	60 seconds	
Stretch and cool down		

Stretch

A strength-training workout always starts with a thorough stretch. Your stretches should target as many areas as possible—legs, arms, back, neck, and butt muscles. Try the following full-body stretch routine. Hold each stretch for 15 seconds.

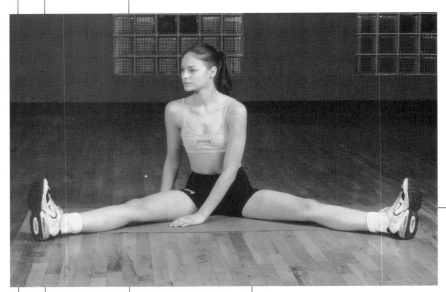

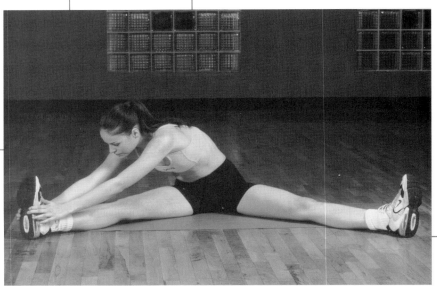

Sitting with legs straight out in a wide straddle, reach down your right side, bringing chest as close to knee as you can. You don't have to be able to touch your feet. Repeat on left side.

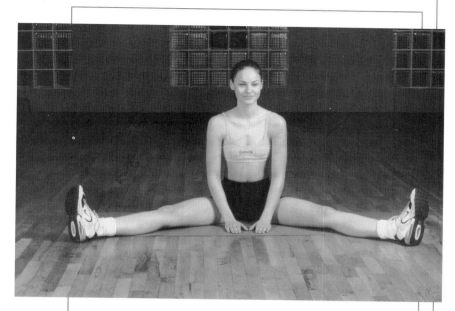

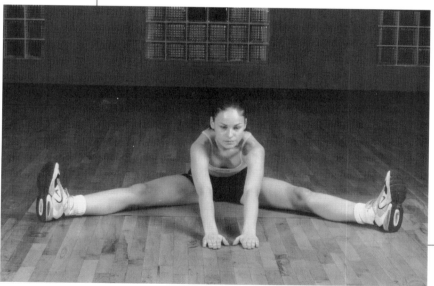

Walk hands up the middle, bringing chest as close to floor between your legs as you can.

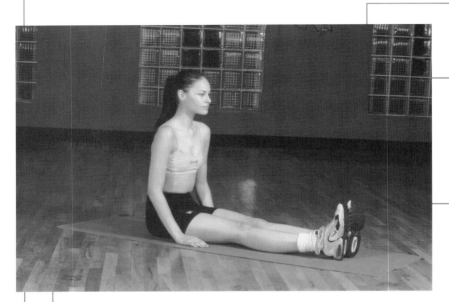

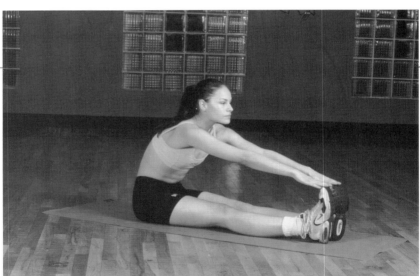

Bring legs together and walk your hands up toward your feet. This is a pike stretch.

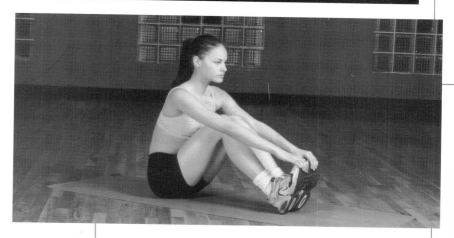

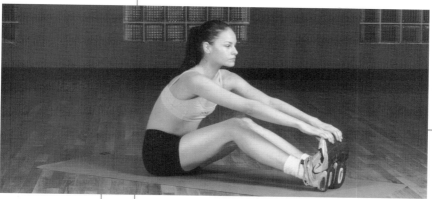

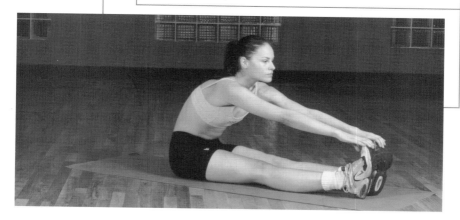

Bring knees up to chest and grab your toes. Straighten legs out as much as you can. Flex your toes and pull back.

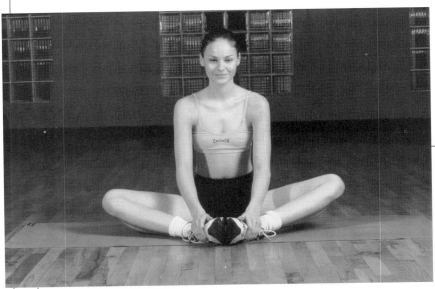

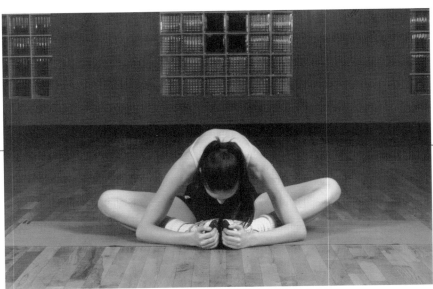

Bring your feet into your middle in a butterfly position. Put your hands on your feet and put your head down.

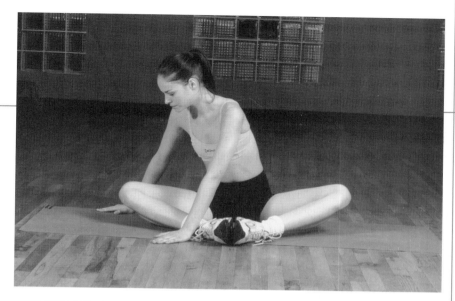

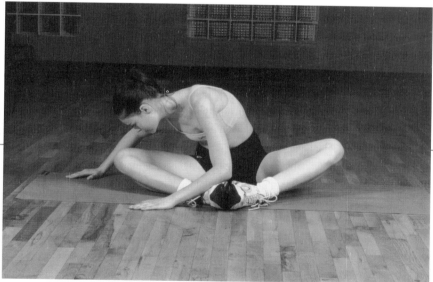

Placing your hands on the floor on either side of your knee, lower your head toward your knee. Repeat on other side.

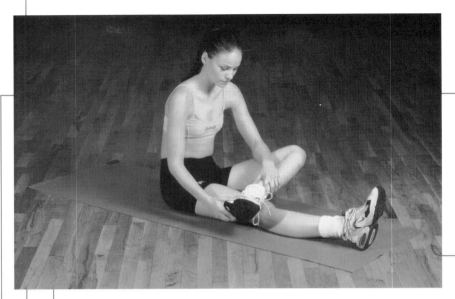

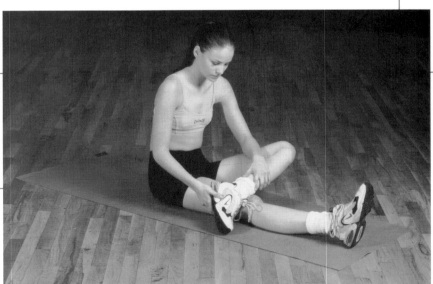

Put one leg out straight and put opposite leg's foot to straight leg's knee. Rotate ankle each way.

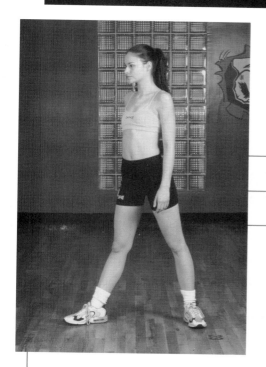

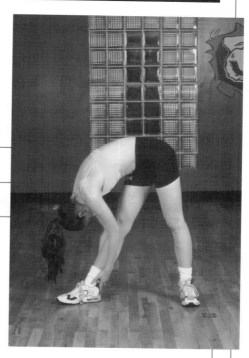

Stand up, with legs apart and feet pointing out. Turn body to the right, making sure your chest is in line with your knee. Work hands down your right side to your feet. Repeat on left side.

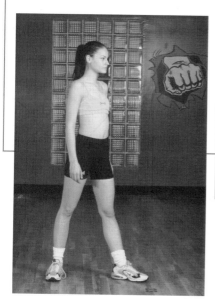

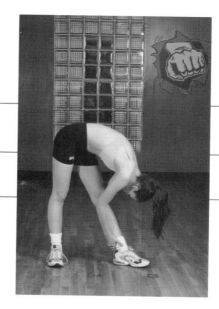

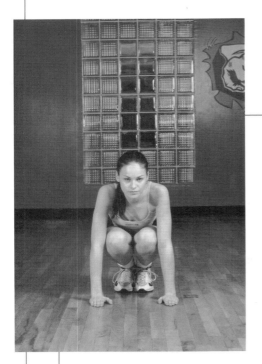

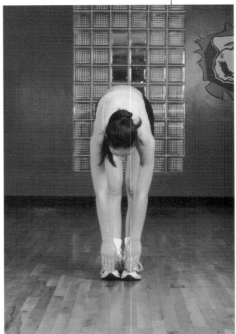

Squat with knees together and place hands on the floor in front of you. Lift your butt up while grasping your toes.

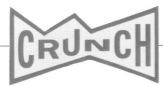

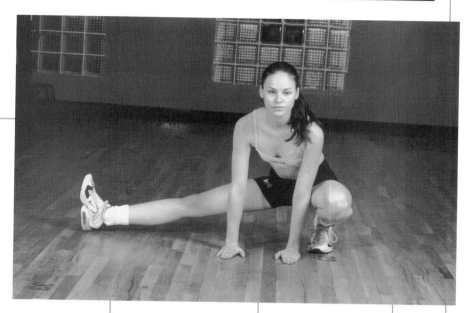

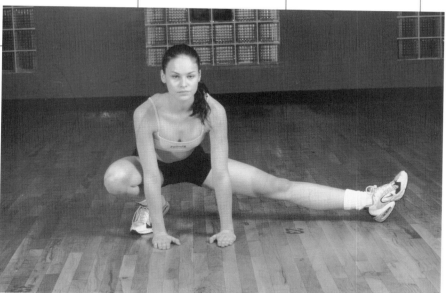

Standing with legs together, squat down. Fully extend right leg, putting hands flat on the floor. Your right heel should touch the ground. Don't hyperextend your knee. Hold for 10 seconds. Repeat on opposite side. Do two sets.

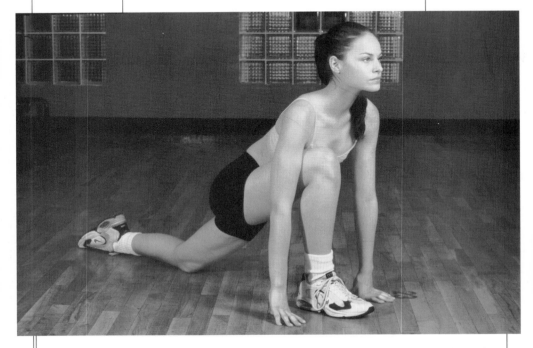

Lunge, putting one knee to the floor. Keep hips square. Put hands down and stretch forward, bringing chest down. Turn heel out. Repeat with opposite leg.

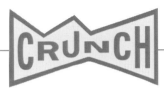

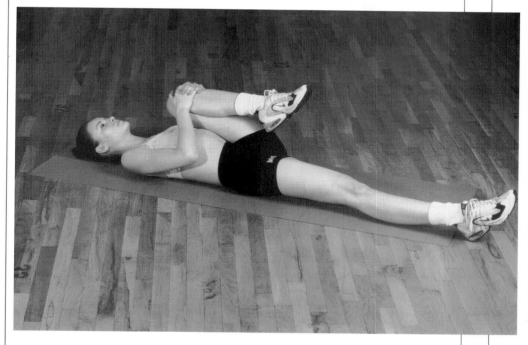

Lie on your back. Pull one leg up in to your chest. Repeat with other leg.

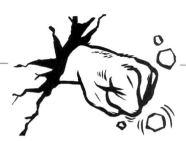

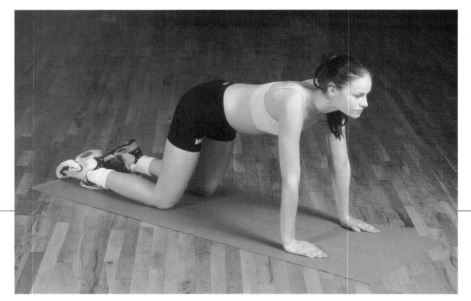

On all fours, bring your head down to the ground and stretch your arms out. This is a cat stretch.

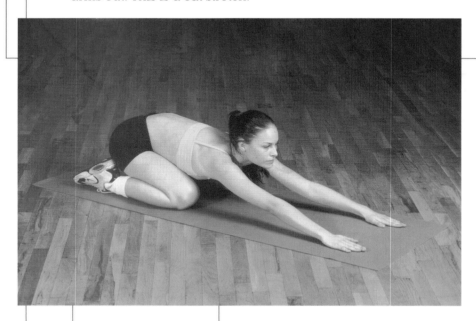

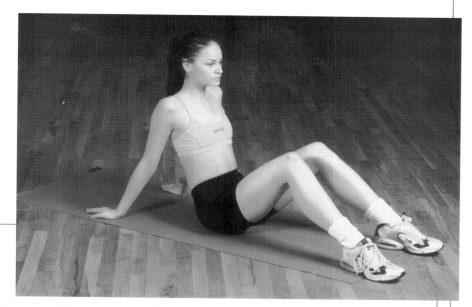

Flip over. With arms shoulder-length apart, hands on the floor with fingers pointing back, lift shoulders off ground and raise knees, keeping feet on floor. Keep your chest up. This is an M stretch.

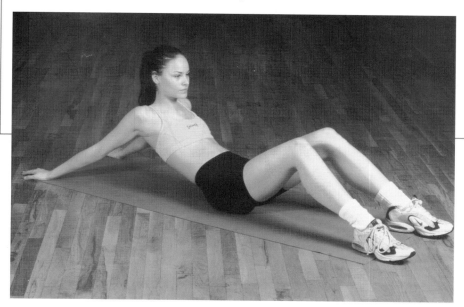

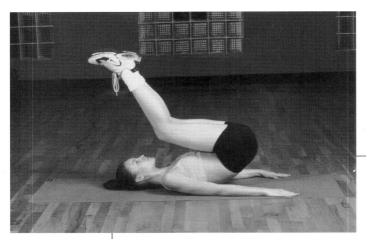

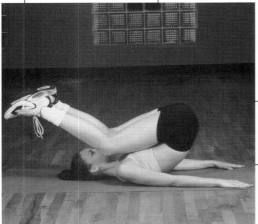

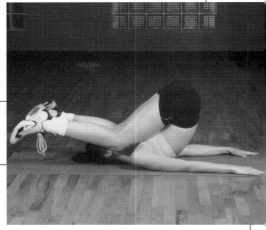

Lie down flat on your back. Kick legs over your head. Straddle your head, touch knees to the ground. Slowly roll legs back to the ground. Do twice.

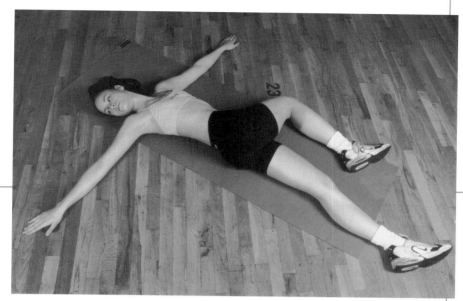

Lie flat on your back, with arms straight out to sides. Cross one leg over the other and turn head to look at opposite arm. Alternate sides. This is a good glute stretch. For a deeper stretch, change the height of the knee.

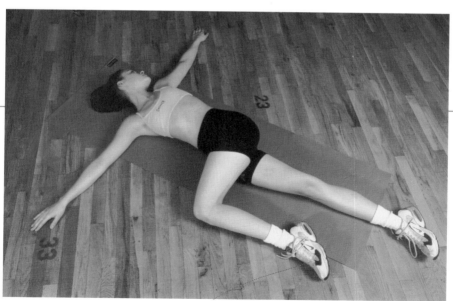

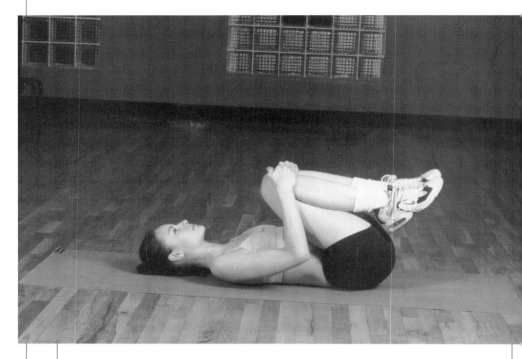

Lie on your back, grab your knees and pull them up to your chest.

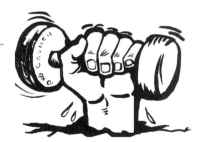

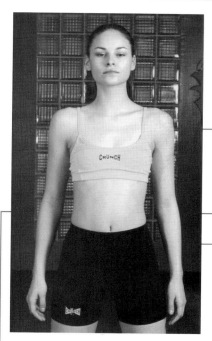
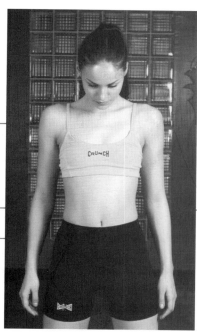

Do neck circles, but do not grind your neck *back*—it may damage your cartilage.

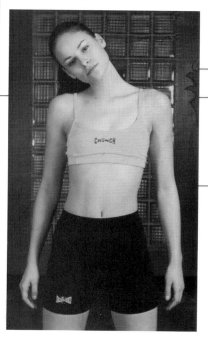
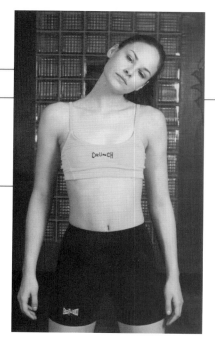

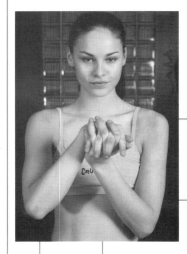

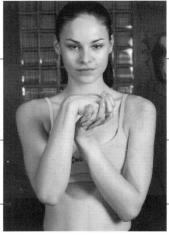

Clasp your hands together and rotate your wrist in circles.

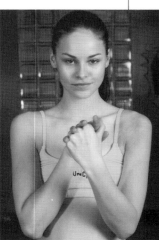

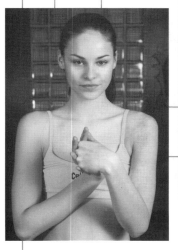

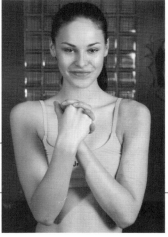

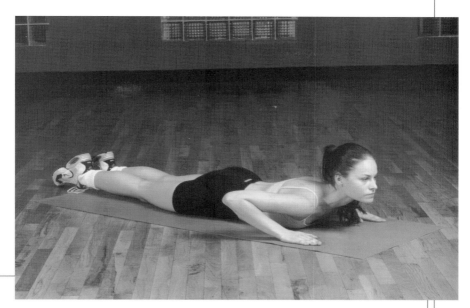

Lie on your stomach in the push-up position, and slowly push your chest up. Keep your hips on the ground and your neck back. This is a seal stretch.

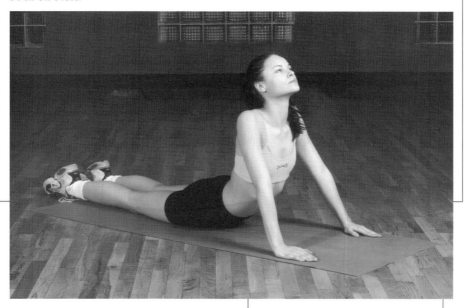

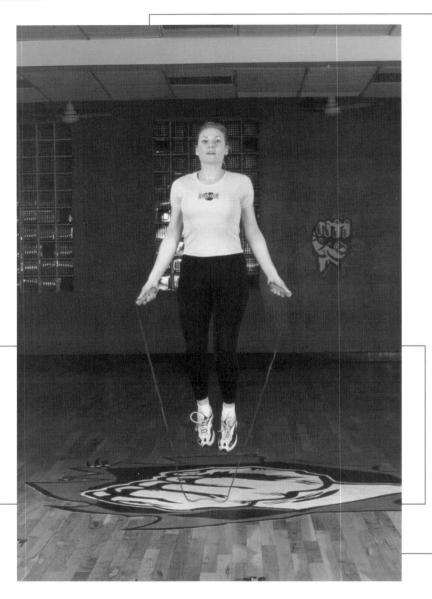

60-SECOND ROPE SKIP/60-SECOND BREAK/
60-SECOND ROPE SKIP:

This routine elevates the heart rate. If a rope is unavailable, or if you lack coordination, jumping jacks can serve as a good alternative.

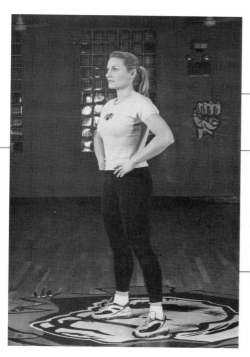

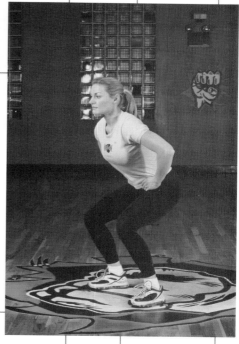

BODY SQUATS:

This is an excellent exercise that targets the thighs and glutes. Place your feet shoulder-width apart and place your hands on your hips. Lower your body toward the floor until your thighs are parallel to the floor and then return to a standing position. Repeat 15 times.

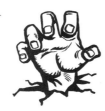

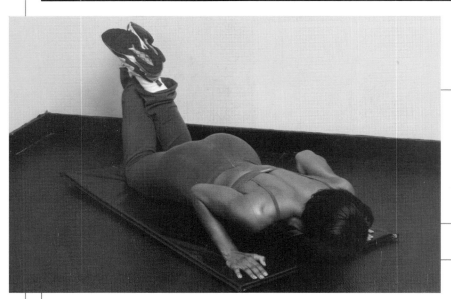

KNEE PUSH-UPS:

Push-ups condition the pectoral (chest) muscles. To begin, lay flat on the floor and place your hands shoulder-width apart. The shoulder blades should be slightly retracted or pinched together. Press your body to a near straight-armed position and lower your body down slowly. Keep your abdominal muscles tight to stabilize the neutral alignment of your body.

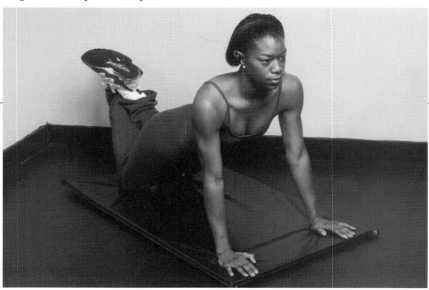

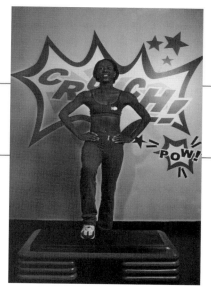
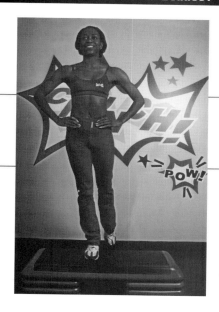

STEP-UPS:

These are done on steps or stairs or with a flat bench surface. The step should be no higher than your knees. One foot should be elevated on the step, while the second foot stays flat on the floor. After a slight push off from the lower leg, the top leg extends from a near right angle (shin and thigh) to an almost straight leg. **Trainer tip:** Don't lock the knee!

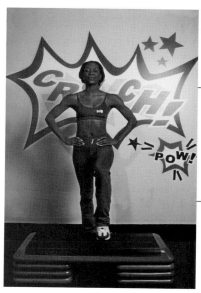
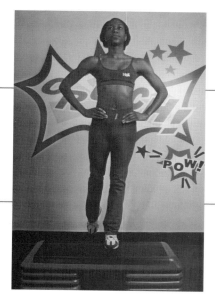

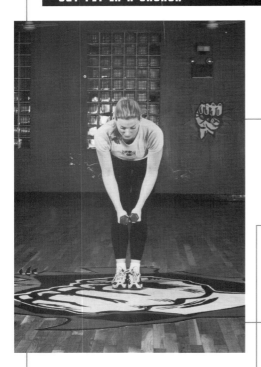

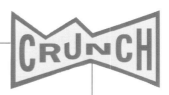

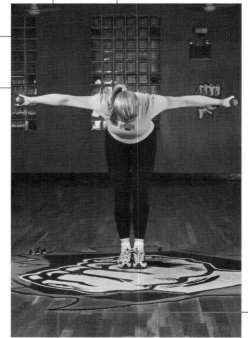

BENT-OVER REAR DELT RAISES:

Standing with knees soft, legs shoulder-width apart, bend from the waist to form a 45 degree angle. Your arms should be slightly bent and hands should grip the dumbbells with palms facing down, holding the weights at knee level. Lifting from the back muscles, raise your arms to shoulder height slowly, then return to starting position. Do not let your arms move behind your shoulders. Keep them in a straight line, making a T with your body.

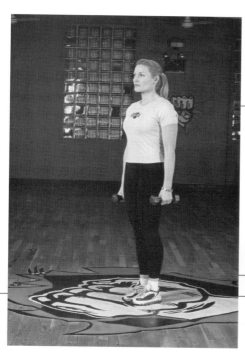

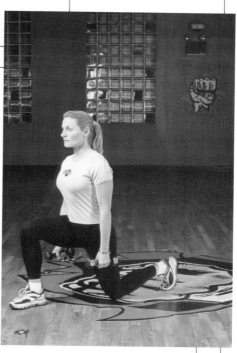

STATIONARY LUNGES (ALSO KNOWN AS ONE-LEGGED SQUATS):

Standing with legs shoulder-width apart and knees soft, take a step approximately 1.5 times your normal stride forward. Raise the heel of the back leg up so that you're standing on the balls of your foot. From this position, keeping the upper body over the torso, bend the back leg, bringing its knee to the ground. Raise up and repeat.

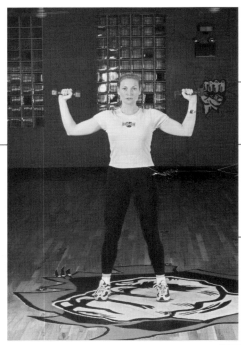

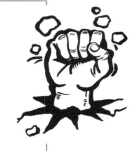

OVERHEAD SHOULDER DUMBBELL PRESS (USING 5 LB. WEIGHTS):

Stand with your feet shoulder-width apart. With your arms at your sides and elbows bent, lift the dumbbells over your head.

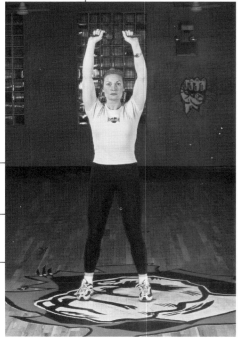

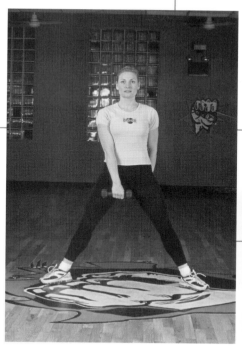

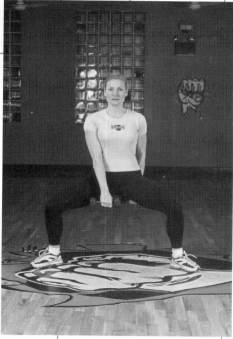

PLIÉ SQUATS:

With your toes pointing outward and heels just outside shoulder-width apart, hold one dumbbell in front of your body and the other in back of your body. Keep your glutes tight and lower your butt until your lower legs and thighs are at right angles. Raise back up and avoid locking your knees.

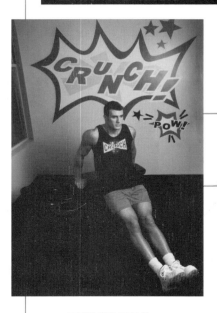 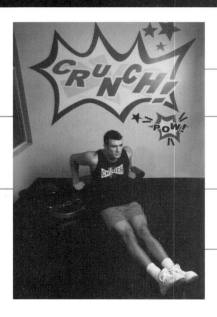

BENCH DIPS:

Sit on the edge of a chair or bench and grasp the seat of the chair on either side of your hips. Keep your knees straight (or bent for an easier dip) and keep your weight on your heels, while lowering your butt toward the floor. Raise back up. Keep your back flat against the chair.

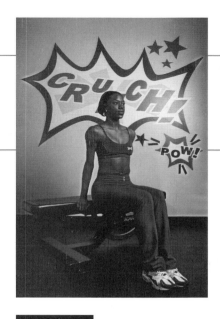 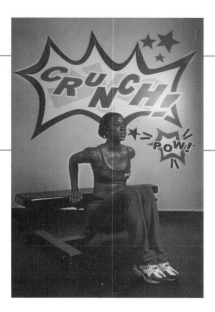

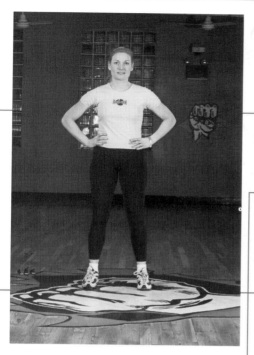

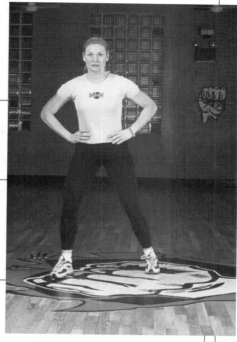

SIDE STEPS:

Stand up with your feet shoulder-width apart, knees soft, and hands on your hips. Draw an imaginary line in front of your toes. Step to the side, placing the heel of the extended leg just in front of the line while bending at the extended knee. Inhale while returning to the starting position. Repeat with other leg. **Trainer tip**: Make sure the knee doesn't extend past the toe when you're taking that side step.

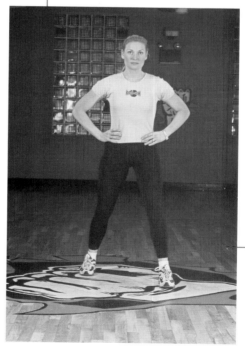

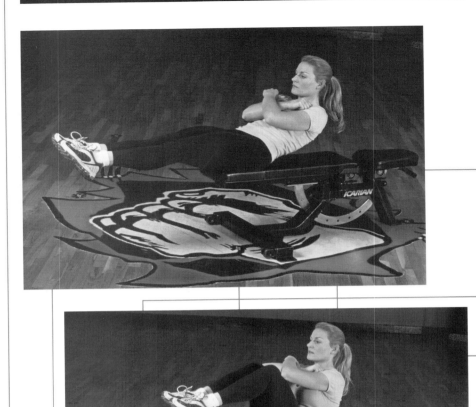

ABDOMINAL CLAMS:

Clams are an excellent abdominal exercise because they recruit both lower and upper abdominal muscles. Begin with your hands behind your neck (or across your chest), your knees bent, and your feet elevated. Curl the upper body up and draw the knees into the body at the same time. **Trainer tip:** Be sure to avoid pulling in the neck!

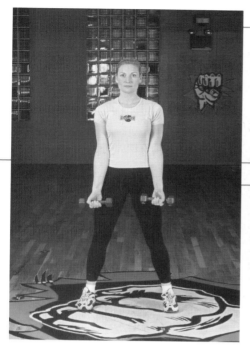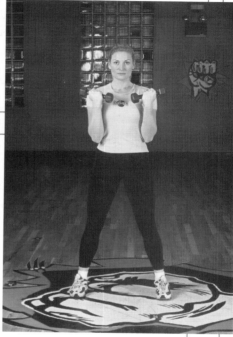

DUMBBELL CURL (USING 5 LB. WEIGHTS):

With your arms at your sides and your palms facing up, lift the dumbbells to your shoulders.

60-SECOND ROPE SKIP/60-SECOND BREAK/ 60-SECOND ROPE SKIP.

STRETCH AND COOL DOWN.

You've made it through your first tough workout!

DAY 3

We're going to step up the pace a bit, and ask you to jog for four minutes, then walk for 16. Stretch out before and after . . . go enjoy the day!

DAY 4

Today, we repeat what we learned in Day 2 but challenge the body by working 1½ circuits. Our ultimate goal is to complete two full circuits.

Exercise	Reps / Time / Weight	
Warm-up	10–15 minutes	
Warm up/Stretch		
Jump rope	60 seconds	
Break	30 seconds	
Jump rope	60 seconds	
Body squats	1 set of 15	
Knee push-ups	1 set of 15	
Step-ups	1 set of 15 per leg	
Bent-over, seated rear deltoid raises	1 set of 15	5 lbs
Break	20 seconds	
Stationary lunges	1 set of 15 per leg	
Overhead shoulder presses	1 set of 15	
Plié squats	1 set of 15	
Bench tricep dips	1 set of 12	
Side steps	1 set of 20 per leg	
Dumbbell curls	1 set of 15	5–8 lbs.
Abdominal clams	2 sets of 10–25	
Jump rope	60 seconds	
Break	30 seconds	
Jump rope	60 seconds	
Squats	1 set of 15	
Knee push-ups	1 set of 15	
Step-ups	1 set of 15	
Bent-over, seated rear delt raises	1 set of 15	5 lbs.
Stationary lunges	1 set of 15 per leg	
Overhead dumbbell shoulder presses	1 set of 15	5 lbs.
Abdominal clams	2 sets of 10–25	
Jump rope	60 seconds	
Stretch and cool down		

DAY 5

Today's cardio workout is an eight-minute jog followed by a 12-minute walk.

DAY 6

Today, you'll complete two full circuits.

Exercise	Reps / Time / Weight	
Warm up/Stretch		
Jump rope	90 seconds	
Squats	1 set of 15	
Knee push-ups	1 set of 15	
Step-ups	1 set of 15 per leg	
Bent-over, seated rear deltoid raises	1 set of 15	5 lbs.
Stationary lunges	1 set of 15 per leg	
Overhead shoulder presses	1 set of 15	
Plié squats	1 set of 15	
Bench tricep dips	1 set of 12	
Side steps	1 set of 20 per leg	
Dumbbell curls	1 set of 15	5–8 lbs.
Abdominal clams	1 set of 25	
Jump rope	90 seconds	
Squats	1 set of 15	
Knee push-ups	1 set of 15	
Step-ups	1 set of 15	
Bent-over, seated rear delt raises	1 set of 15	5 lbs.
Stationary lunges	1 set of 15 per leg	
Overhead dumbbell shoulder presses	1 set of 15	5 lbs.
Plié squats	1 set of 15	
Bench dips	1 set of 12	
Side steps	1 set of 20 each leg	
Dumbbell curls	1 set of 15	5–8 lbs.
Abdominal clams	1 set of 25	
Jump rope	90 seconds	
Stretch and cool down		

DAY 7

Rest . . . relax . . . enjoy!

WEEK 2

DAY 1

Take a 12-minute jog and an eight-minute walk.

DAY 2

Exercise	Reps / Time / Weight	
Warm up/Stretch		
Jump rope	2 minutes	
Squats	1 set of 15	
Straight-leg push-ups	1 set of 5	
Knee push-ups	1 set of 10	
Step-ups	1 set of 15 per leg	
Bent-over, seated rear deltoid raises	1 set of 15	8 lbs.
Stationary lunges	1 set of 15 per leg	5 lbs.
Overhead shoulder presses	1 set of 15	8 lbs.
Plié squats	1 set of 15	5 lbs.
Bench dips	1 set of 15	
Side steps	1 set of 25 per leg	
Dumbbell curls	1 set of 15	8 lbs.
Abdominal clams	1 set of 25	

Note: *You're now at the half-way point between the circuits. You'll see in the second round, you'll be increasing the difficulty of the workout.*

Jump rope	2 minutes	
Squats	1 set of 15	
Knee push-ups	1 set of 15	
Step-ups	1 set of 15	
Bent-over, seated rear delt raises	1 set of 15	5 lbs.
Stationary lunges	1 set of 15 per leg	
Overhead dumbbell shoulder presses	1 set of 15	5 lbs.
Plié squats	1 set of 15	
Bench dips	1 set of 12	
Side steps	1 set of 20 each leg	
Dumbbell curls	1 set of 15	8 lbs.
Abdominal clams	1 set of 25	
Jump rope	2 minutes	
Stretch and cool down		

DAY 3

Jog for 16 minutes, then walk for four.

DAY 4

Exercise	Reps / Time / Weight	
Warm up/Stretch		
Jump rope	2 minutes	
Jumping jacks	25	
Squats	1 set of 15	5 lbs.
Straight-leg push-ups	5	
Knee push-ups	10	
Step-ups	1 set of 15 per leg	5 lbs.
Bent-over, seated rear deltoid raises	1 set of 15	8 lbs.
Stationary lunges	1 set of 15 per leg	5 lbs.
Overhead shoulder presses	1 set of 15	8 lbs.
Plié squats	1 set of 15	5 lbs.
Bench dips	1 set of 15	
Side steps	1 set of 25 per leg	
Dumbbell curls	1 set of 15	8 lbs.
Abdominal clams	1 set of 25	
Jump rope	2 minutes	
Squats	1 set of 15	5 lbs.
Straight-leg push-ups	5	
Knee push-ups	10	
Step-ups	1 set of 15	5 lbs.
Bent-over, seated rear delt raises	1 set of 15	8 lbs.
Stationary lunges	1 set of 15 per leg	5 lbs.
Overhead dumbbell shoulder presses	1 set of 15	8 lbs.
Plié squats	1 set of 15	5 lbs.
Bench dips	1 set of 15	
Side steps	1 set of 25 each leg	
Dumbbell curls	1 set of 15	8 lbs.
Abdominal clams	1 set of 25	
Jump rope	2 minutes	
Stretch and cool down		

DAY 5

Jog for 20 minutes.

DAY 6

Exercise	Reps / Time / Weight	
Warm up/StretchJump rope	2 minutes	
Jumping jacks	25	
Squats	1 set of 15	8 lbs.
Straight-leg push-ups	10	
Knee push-ups	5	
Step-ups	1 set of 15 per leg	8 lbs.
Bent-over, seated rear deltoid raises	1 set of 15	10 lbs.
Stationary lunges	1 set of 15 per leg	8 lbs.
Overhead shoulder presses	1 set of 15	10 lbs.
Plié squats	1 set of 15	8 lbs.
Bench dips	1 set of 20	
Side steps	1 set of 30 per leg	
Dumbbell curls	1 set of 15	10 lbs.
Abdominal clams	1 set of 25	
Jump rope	2 minutes	
Squats	1 set of 15	5 lbs.
Straight-leg push-ups	5	
Knee push-ups	10	
Step-ups	1 set of 15	5 lbs.
Bent-over, seated rear delt raises	1 set of 15	8 lbs.
Stationary lunges	1 set of 15 per leg	5 lbs.
Overhead dumbbell shoulder presses	1 set of 15	8 lbs.
Plié squats	1 set of 15	5 lbs.
Bench dips	1 set of 15	
Side steps	1 set of 25 each leg	
Dumbbell curls	1 set of 15	8 lbs.
Abdominal clams	1 set of 25	
Jump rope	2 minutes	
Stretch and cool down		

DAY 7

Enjoy your day of rest!

WEEK 3

For the next two weeks, you'll be changing your method of cardio-vascular exercise. You'll be starting what's called Interval Cardio Workouts. This is a way to combat the body's natural inclination to plateau. By shaking up the system, the body won't adjust to a routine and thus will be tricked into shape.

Each of the cardio-training days in these weeks will be slightly different. Because the body reaches plateaus quickly, CRUNCH's cardio-training philosophy incorporates three different routines in order to keep your body guessing by varying the intensity of the workout. This will help increase your aerobic capacity, which allows your body to burn calories more efficiently and with greater speed.

Here are the three stages of interval cardiovascular training:

1. Twenty-four minutes on cardiovascular equipment, rotating in six, two-minute intervals—for a total of six intervals of high intensity and six intervals of low intensity. For example, if you normally jog on the treadmill at a speed of 6.0, rotate in six, two-minute intervals sprinting at 8.0 for two minutes, then 6.0, then 8.0, etc. Today, you will have a shorter workout, but use 50% of your time at a high intensity.

2. Thirty-six minutes on the cardiovascular machine, again rotating six, two-minute intervals at a high intensity (e.g., four minutes at 6.0, then two minutes at 8.0, etc.). When you reach this step, you will operate at a 3:1 ratio of high intensity to your normal pace.

3. Forty-eight minutes on the cardiovascular machine, rotating six, two-minute intervals at a high intensity (e.g., six minutes at 6.0, then two minutes at 8.0).

DAY 1

Start the week with the 24-minute interval jog.

DAY 2

Exercise	Reps / Time / Weight	
Stretch		
Jump rope	2 minutes	
Jumping jacks	25	
Squats	1 set of 15	8 lbs.
Straight-leg push-ups	10	
Knee push-ups	5	
Step-ups	1 set of 15 per leg	8 lbs.
Bent-over, seated rear deltoid raises	1 set of 15	10 lbs.
Stationary lunges	1 set of 15 per leg	8 lbs.
Overhead shoulder presses	1 set of 15	10 lbs.
Plié squats	1 set of 15	8 lbs.
Bench dips	1 set of 20	
Side steps	1 set of 30 per leg	
Dumbbell curls	1 set of 15	10 lbs.
Abdominal clams	1 set of 25	
Jump rope	2 minutes	
Jumping jacks	25	
Squats	1 set of 15	8 lbs.
Straight-leg push-ups	10	
Knee push-ups	5	
Step-ups	1 set of 15	8 lbs.
Bent-over, seated rear delt raises	1 set of 15	10 lbs.
Stationary lunges	1 set of 15 per leg	8 lbs.
Overhead dumbbell shoulder presses	1 set of 15	10 lbs.
Plié squats	1 set of 15	8 lbs.
Bench dips	1 set of 20	
Side steps	1 set of 30 each leg	
Dumbbell curls	1 set of 15	10 lbs.
Abdominal clams	1 set of 25	
Jump rope	2 minutes	
Stretch and cool down		

DAY 3

Go for a 28-minute jog.

DAY 4

Exercise	Reps / Time / Weight	
Warm up/Stretch		
Jump rope	2 minutes	
Jumping jacks	50	
Squats	1 set of 15	10 lbs.
Straight-leg push-ups	15	
Step-ups	1 set of15 per leg	10 lbs.
Bent-over, seated rear deltoid raises	1 set of 15	10 lbs.
Bent-over, seated rear deltoid raises	1 set of 15	5 lbs.
Stationary lunges	1 set of 15 per leg	10 lbs.
Overhead shoulder presses	1 set of 15	10 lbs.
Overhead shoulder presses	1 set of 15	5 lbs.
Plié squats	1 set of 15	10 lbs.
Bench dips	1 set of 20	
Dumbbell kickbacks	1 set of 15	
Side steps	1 set of 35 per leg	
Dumbbell curls	1 set of 15	10 lbs.
Dumbbell curls	1 set of 15	5 lbs.
Abdominal clams	1 set of 25	
Jump rope	2 minutes	
Jumping jacks	25	
Squats	1 set of 15	8 lbs.
Straight-leg push-ups	10	
Knee push-ups	5	
Step-ups	1 set of 15	8 lbs.
Bent-over, seated rear delt raises	1 set of 15	10 lbs.
Stationary lunges	1 set of 15 per leg	8 lbs.
Overhead dumbbell shoulder presses	1 set of 15	10 lbs.
Plié squats	1 set of 15	8 lbs.
Bench dips	1 set of 20	
Side steps	1 set of 30 each leg	
Dumbbell curls	1 set of 15	10 lbs.
Abdominal clams	1 set of 25	
Jump rope	2 minutes	
Stretch and cool down		

You'll notice there's a new move in this day's workout:

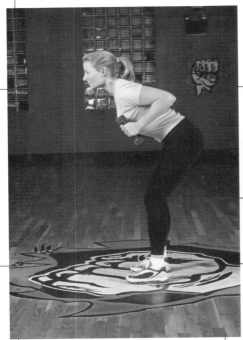

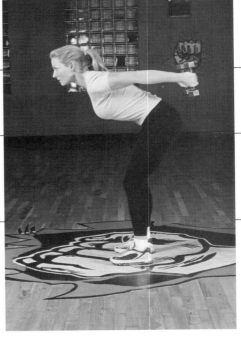

TRICEP KICKBACKS:

Stand with feet shoulder-width apart. Keeping knees soft, bend forward straight back from the waist to a 45 degree angle. Gripping the weights with your palms facing in, keep the elbows close to the body. From the back of the arm, raise your elbows just past your back. This is your starting position. Now, exhale while extending the full arm behind your body, bringing the arm into a straight position. Hold for two counts and release slowly, bringing weights back to starting position. Concentrate on squeezing the tricep and feeling the muscle!

DAY 5

Today, take a 32-minute jog.

DAY 6

Exercise	Reps / Time / Weight	
Warm up/Stretch		
Jump rope	2 minutes	
Jumping jacks	50	
Squats	1 set of 15	10 lbs.
Straight-leg push-ups	15	
Step-ups	1 set of 15 per leg	10 lbs.
Bent-over, seated rear deltoid raises	1 set of 15	10 lbs.
Bent-over, seated rear deltoid raises	1 set of 15	5 lbs.
Stationary lunges	1 set of 15 per leg	10 lbs.
Overhead shoulder presses	1 set of 15	10 lbs.
Overhead shoulder presses	1 set of 15	5 lbs.
Plié squats	1 set of 15	10 lbs.
Bench dips	1 set of 20	
Dumbbell kickbacks	1 set of 15	5 lbs.
Side steps	1 set of 35 per leg	
Dumbbell curls	1 set of 15	10 lbs.
Dumbbell curls	1 set of 15	5 lbs.
Abdominal clams	1 set of 25	
Jump rope	2 minutes	
Jumping jacks	25	
Squats	1 set of 15	10 lbs.
Straight-leg push-ups	15	
Step-ups	1 set of 15 per leg	10 lbs.
Bent-over, seated rear deltoid raises	1 set of 15	10 lbs.
Bent-over, seated rear deltoid raises	1 set of 15	5 lbs.
Stationary lunges	1 set of 15 per leg	10 lbs.
Overhead shoulder presses	1 set of 15	10 lbs.
Overhead shoulder presses	1 set of 15	5 lbs.
Plié squats	1 set of 15	10 lbs.
Bench dips	1 set of 20	
Dumbbell kickbacks	1 set of 15	5 lbs.
Side steps	1 set of 35 per leg	
Dumbbell curls	1 set of 15	10 lbs.
Dumbbell curls	1 set of 15	5 lbs.
Abdominal clams	1 set of 25	
Jump rope	2 minutes	
Jumping jacks	25	
Stretch and cool down		

DAY 7

Rest!

WEEK 4

DAY 1

Go for a 34-minute jog.

DAY 2

Exercise	Reps / Time / Weight	
Warm up/Stretch		
Jump rope	2 minutes	
Jumping jacks	50	
Squats	1 set of 15	10 lbs.
Step-ups	1 set of 15 per leg	10 lbs.
Straight-leg push-ups	15	
Bent-over, seated rear deltoid raises	1 set of 15	10 lbs.
Bent-over, seated rear deltoid raises	1 set of 15	5 lbs.
Stationary lunges	1 set of 15 per leg	10 lbs.
Overhead shoulder presses	1 set of 15	10 lbs.
Overhead shoulder presses	1 set of 15	5 lbs.
Plié squats	1 set of 15	10 lbs.
Side steps	1 set of 35 per leg	
Bench dips	1 set of 20	
Dumbbell kickbacks	1 set of 15	5 lbs.
Dumbbell curls	1 set of 15	10 lbs.
Dumbbell curls	1 set of 15	5 lbs.
Abdominal clams	1 set of 25	
Jump rope	2 minutes	
Jumping jacks	50	
Squats	1 set of 15	10 lbs.
Straight-leg push-ups	15	
Step-ups	1 set of 15 per leg	10 lbs.
Bent-over, seated rear deltoid raises	1 set of 15	10 lbs.
Bent-over, seated rear deltoid raises	1 set of 15	5 lbs.
Stationary lunges	1 set of 15 per leg	10 lbs.
Overhead shoulder presses	1 set of 15	10 lbs.
Overhead shoulder presses	1 set of 15	5 lbs.
Plié squats	1 set of 15	10 lbs.
Bench dips	1 set of 20	
Dumbbell kickbacks	1 set of 15	5 lbs.
Side steps	1 set of 35 per leg	
Dumbbell curls	1 set of 15	10 lbs.

DAY 2 (continued)

Exercise	Reps / Time / Weight	
Dumbbell curls	1 set of 15	5 lbs.
Abdominal clams	1 set of 25	
Jump rope	2 minutes	
Jumping jacks	50	
Stretch and cool down		

DAY 3

Go for a 38-minute interval jog.

DAY 4

Exercise	Reps / Time / Weight	
Warm up/Stretch		
Jump rope	2 minutes	
Jumping jacks	50	
Squats	1 set of 15	10 lbs.
Step-ups	1 set of 15 per leg	10 lbs.
Straight-leg push-ups	15	
Bent-over, seated rear deltoid raises	1 set of 15	10 lbs.
Bent-over, seated rear deltoid raises	1 set of 15	5 lbs.
Stationary lunges	1 set of 15 per leg	10 lbs.
Overhead shoulder presses	1 set of 15	10 lbs.
Overhead shoulder presses	1 set of 15	8 lbs.
Plié squats	1 set of 15	10 lbs.
Side steps	1 set of 35 per leg	
Bench dips	1 set of 20	
Dumbbell kickbacks	1 set of 15	5 lbs.
Dumbbell curls	1 set of 15	10 lbs.
Dumbbell curls	1 set of 15	5 lbs.
Abdominal clams	1 set of 25	
Jump rope	2 minutes	
Jumping jacks	50	
Squats	1 set of 15	10 lbs.
Step-ups	1 set of 15 per leg	
Step-ups	1 set of 15 per leg	
Straight-leg push-ups	15	
Bent-over, seated rear deltoid raises	1 set of 15	10 lbs.
Bent-over, seated rear deltoid raises	1 set of 15	5 lbs.
Stationary lunges	1 set of 15 per leg	10 lbs.
Overhead shoulder presses	1 set of 15	10 lbs.

DAY 4 (continued)

Exercise	Reps / Time / Weight	
Overhead shoulder presses	1 set of 15	5 lbs.
Plié squats	1 set of 15	10 lbs.
Side steps	1 set of 35 per leg	
Bench dips	1 set of 20	
Dumbbell kickbacks	1 set of 15	5 lbs.
Dumbbell curls	1 set of 15	10 lbs.
Dumbbell curls	1 set of 15	5 lbs.
Abdominal clams	1 set of 25	
Jump rope	2 minutes	
Jumping jacks	50	
Stretch and cool down		

DAY 5

Take a 42-minute jog. Although this is the last cardio workout in the Four-Week Workout, you should consider extending your cardio workouts for another two days to reach the third stage of interval training: the 48-minute interval jog. That means the next cardio day's jog would be for 44 minutes, and the following one for 48 minutes, in intervals.

DAY 6

Exercise	Reps / Time / Weight	
Warm up/Stretch		
Jump rope	2 minutes	
Jumping jacks	50	
Squats	1 set of 15	10 lbs.
Step-ups	1 set of 15 per leg	10 lbs.
Straight-leg push-ups	15	
Bent-over, seated rear deltoid raises	1 set of 15	10 lbs.
Bent-over, seated rear deltoid raises	1 set of 15	5 lbs.
Stationary lunges	1 set of 15 per leg	10 lbs.
Overhead shoulder presses	1 set of 15	10 lbs.
Overhead shoulder presses	1 set of 15	8 lbs.
Plié squats	1 set of 15	10 lbs.
Side steps	1 set of 35 per leg	
Bench dips	1 set of 20	
Dumbbell kickbacks	1 set of 15	5 lbs.
Dumbbell curls	1 set of 15	10 lbs.

DAY 6 [continued]

Exercise	Reps / Time / Weight	
Dumbbell curls	1 set of 15	5 lbs.
Abdominal clams	1 set of 25	
Jump rope	2 minutes	
Jumping jacks	50	
Squats	1 set of 15	10 lbs.
Step-ups	1 set of 15 per leg	
Step-ups	1 set of 15 per leg	
Straight-leg push-ups	15	
Bent-over, seated rear deltoid raises	1 set of 15	10 lbs.
Bent-over, seated rear deltoid raises	1 set of 15	5 lbs.
Stationary lunges	1 set of 15 per leg	10 lbs.
Overhead shoulder presses	1 set of 15	10 lbs.
Overhead shoulder presses	1 set of 15	5 lbs.
Plié squats	1 set of 15	10 lbs.
Side steps	1 set of 35 per leg	
Bench dips	1 set of 20	
Dumbbell kickbacks	1 set of 15	5 lbs.
Dumbbell curls	1 set of 15	10 lbs.
Dumbbell curls	1 set of 15	5 lbs.
Abdominal clams	1 set of 25	
Jump rope	2 minutes	
Jumping jacks	50	
Stretch and cool down		

DAY 7

Time to hit the beach!

Carol K. Stewart

PART III
THE 12-WEEK WORKOUT

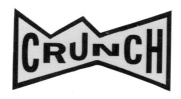

You may think, "Oh, I've got 12 whole weeks to get in shape before the big event!" But you should look at it this way: You've got only three short months!

You can obviously accomplish a lot more in 12 weeks than you can in four, and we've designed the 12-Week Workout to pack as much punch as possible into the time you've got.

You start out with a lower intensity, getting familiar with the exercises and your aerobic capacity. Gradually, you increase the weights on the strength training days and increase your aerobic capacity on the cardio days. You slowly build to complete two full circuits of strength training moves, increasing both weights and reps. And in the final steps of the program, we'll change the approach of the workout to keep your muscles alert and challenged. In fact, this is how the 12-Week Workout differs from the Four-Week Workout, and why merely repeating the Four-Week Workout for 12 weeks isn't as effective: By constantly changing the workout every week—not only changing the kinds of exercises, the repetitions, and weights, but also the order in which you work your muscles—you keep your body guessing and fight its natural tendency to reach a plateau.

STRENGTH TRAINING

Days 1, 3, and 5 of the 12-Week Workout are strength training days. Each workout includes all the major muscle groups. Try to minimize the amount of time between sets. If you need to rest, take no more than 30 seconds to catch your breath and rest your muscles before moving on to the next exercise. Allow an hour for your workouts on these days. Here's a description of exercises you'll be doing.

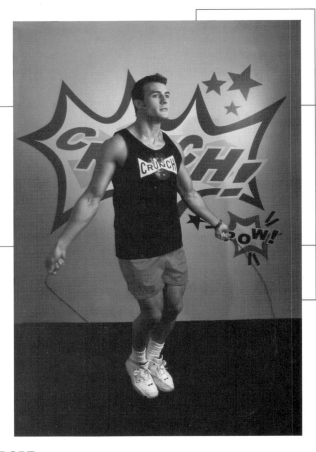

JUMP ROPE:

Not only does jumping rope get your blood pumping, it demands a
certain amount of coordination.

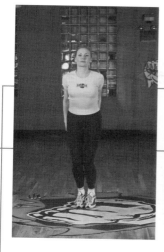

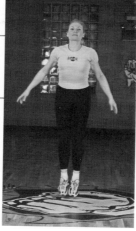

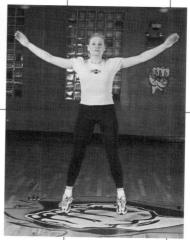

JUMPING JACKS:

To get your workout started, jumping jacks are excellent alternatives to jumping rope and merely running on the treadmill.

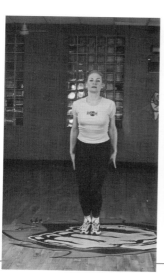

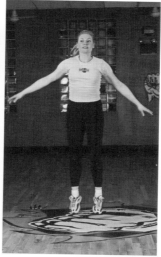

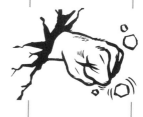

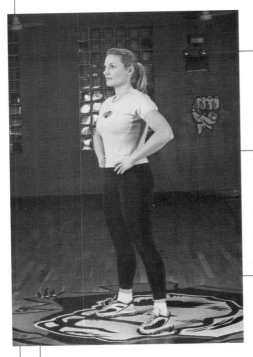

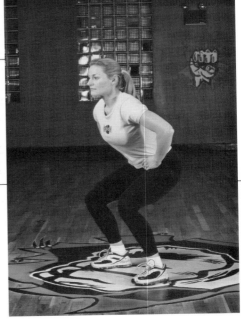

BODY SQUATS:

This is an excellent exercise that targets the hamstrings. Place your feet shoulder-width apart and place your hands on your hips. Lower your body toward the floor until your thighs are parallel to the floor and then return to a standing position.

SQUAT THRUSTS:

Stand straight with your feet shoulder-width apart and knees slightly bent. Imagine you're going to sit in a chair and slowly take your butt back, keeping your spine straight. Bend at the knees into a seated position. While you sit back, extend your arms in front of you for balance. Keep your arms straight and in front of your body while you lift to your standing position. Exhale as you sit, inhale as you stand. **Trainer tip:** While in the seated position, make sure your knees do not go past your toes. This will help you avoid injuring your knees.

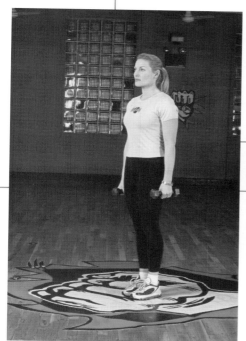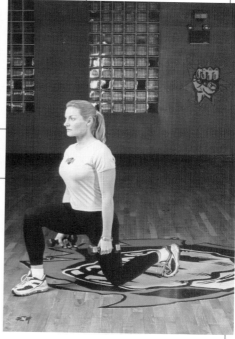

STATIONARY LUNGES:

Standing with legs shoulder-width apart, knees soft, and dumbbells at hip level, take a step approximately 1.5 times your normal stride forward. Raise the heel of the back leg up so that you're standing on the balls of your foot. From this position, keeping the upper body over the torso, bend the back leg, bringing its knee to the ground. Raise up and repeat.

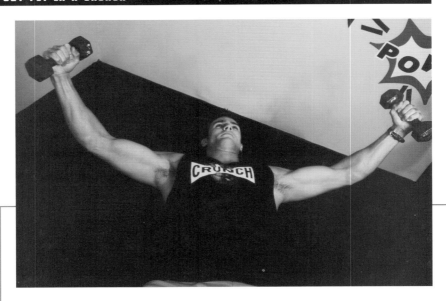

PEC FLIES:

Lie on a bench with dumbbells in your hands, palms facing the ceiling, and arms out to your sides. Create a triangle with your arms and chest—bring your palms slowly up into a "point" above your pectoral muscles. Feel the movement across your chest and not in your arms. Keep your arms in a straight line across your shoulders! The chest muscles should be lifting the weight, *not* the elbows!

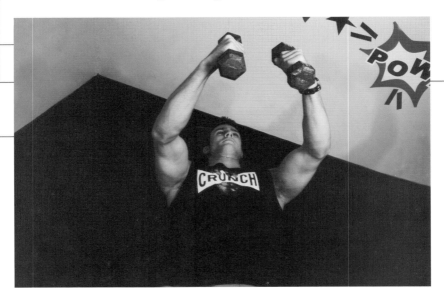

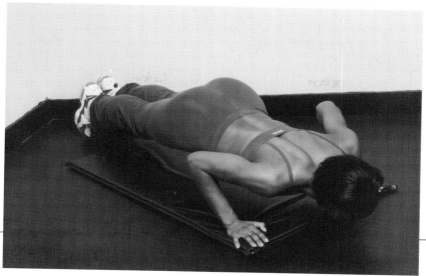

PUSH-UPS:

Push-ups condition the pectoral (chest) muscles. To begin, lay flat on the floor and place your hands shoulder-width apart. The shoulder blades should be slightly retracted or pinched together. Press your body to a near straight-armed position and lower your body down slowly. Keep your abdominal muscles tight to stabilize the neutral alignment of your body. You will start the workouts doing push-ups from the knees, and gradually add straight-leg, or regular, push-ups.

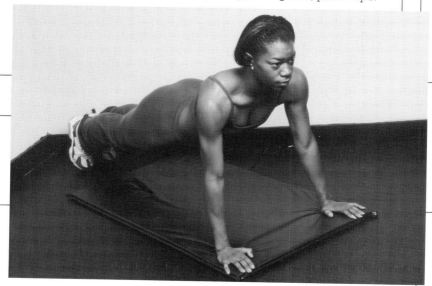

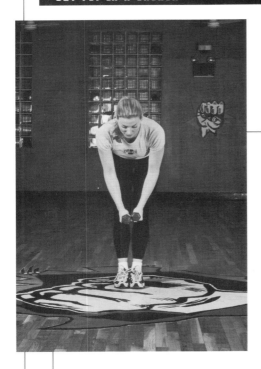

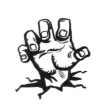

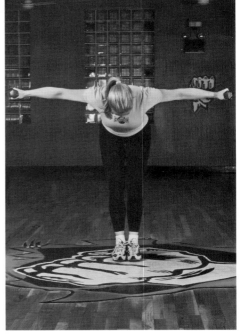

REAR DELT RAISES:

Standing with knees soft, legs shoulder-width apart, bend from the waist to form a 45 degree angle. Your arms should be slightly bent and hands should grip the dumbbells with palms facing down, holding the weights at knee level. Lifting from the back muscles, raise your arms to shoulder height slowly, then return to starting position. Do not let your arms move behind your shoulders. Keep them in a straight line, making a T with your body.

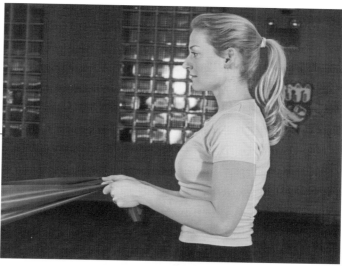

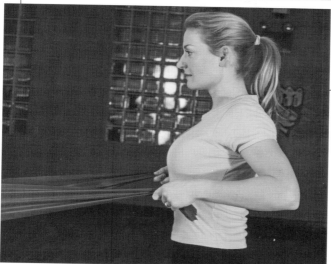

EXERCISE BAND ROWS:

Place the exercise band around a stable pillar or post where you can comfortably hold the ends directly below your chest. Your legs should be shoulder-width apart and your back should be straight and knees soft. Stand far enough from the pillar to achieve moderate tension in the exercise band. Start with the exercise band slightly stretched. Grip the band in both hands, with palms facing each other, and keep your lower body tight and arms close to your body. Draw your elbows and shoulders past the back and squeeze the shoulders into the lateral muscles.

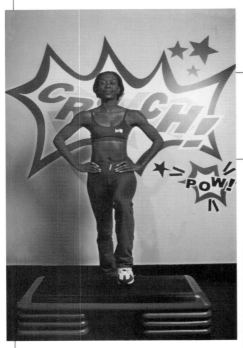

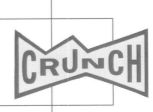

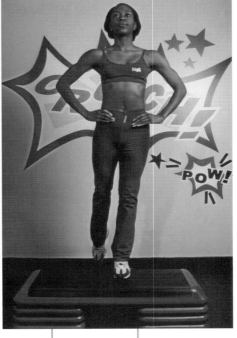

STEP-UPS:

Done on steps or stairs or with a flat bench surface. The step should be no higher than your hips. One foot should be elevated on the step, while the second foot stays flat on the floor. After a slight push off from the lower leg, the top leg extends from a near right angle (shin and thigh) to an almost straight leg. **Trainer tip:** Don't lock the knee!

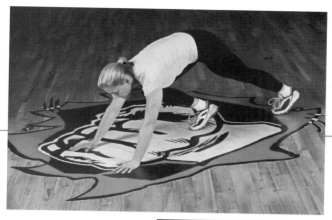

MOUNTAIN CLIMBERS:

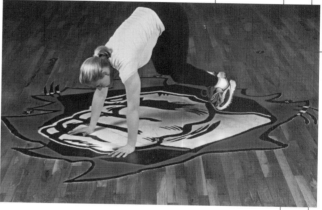

Begin on the floor in the top of the push-up position and bring one knee up to your chest. Keeping a constant motion, alternate pumping your knees into your chest (like a runner's motion). Pay particular attention to keeping your back straight and arms soft enough to absorb shock.

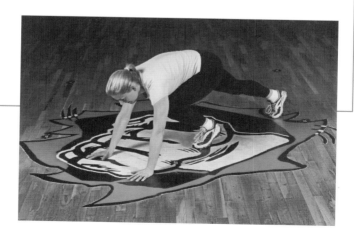

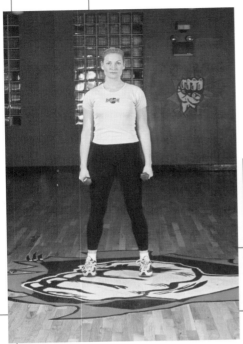

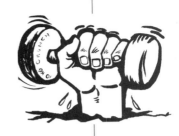

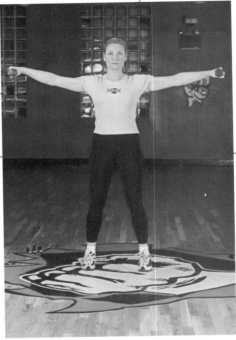

LATERAL RAISES:

Stand straight with your feet shoulder-width apart and knees slightly bent. Grip the dumbbells in your hands with your palms facing down, elbows slightly bent and arms in front of your body. Raise your arms slowly up to the shoulder, exhaling as you do so. Hold for two counts and slowly return to starting position, inhaling slowly. **Trainer's tip:** Use a weight that will allow you to complete the exercise in perfect form, instead of going for the heaviest weight you can carry. Don't take the dumbbell too far over the shoulders, because it will place stress on the shoulders and may injure the rotator cuff.

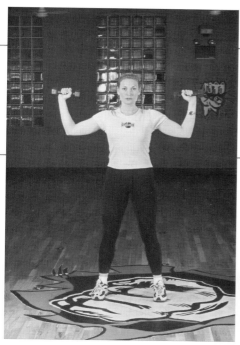

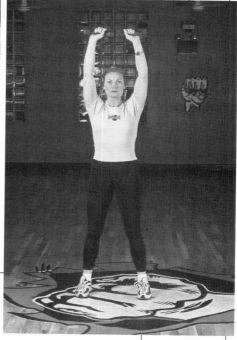

DUMBBELL SHOULDER PRESSES:

Stand with your feet shoulder-width apart. Keep your arms outstretched to your sides, and, as you lift the dumbbells over your head, bend your elbows as they reach shoulder height. This movement pushes the dumbbells toward the ceiling.

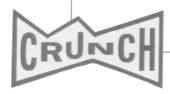

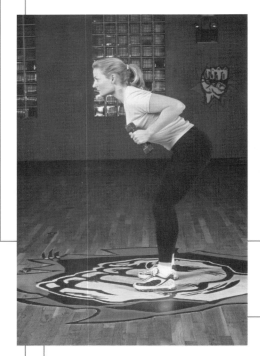

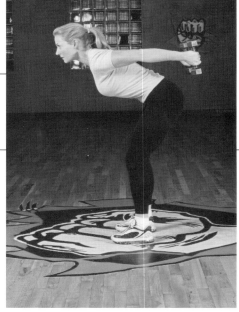

TRICEP KICKBACKS:

Stand with feet shoulder-width apart. Keeping knees soft and back straight, bend forward from the waist to a 45 degree angle. Gripping the weights with your palms facing in, keep the elbows close to the body. From the back of the arm, raise your elbows just past your back. This is your starting position. Now, exhale while extending the full arm behind your body, bringing the arm into a straight position. Hold for two counts and release slowly, bringing weights back to starting position. Concentrate on squeezing the tricep and feeling the muscle!

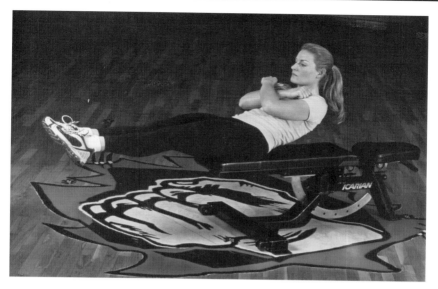

ABDOMINAL CLAMS:

Clams are an excellent abdominal exercise because they recruit both lower and upper abdominal regions. Begin with your hands behind your neck (or across your chest) and keep your knees bent and feet elevated. Curl the upper body up and draw the knees into the body at the same time. **Trainer tip:** Be sure to avoid pulling in the neck!

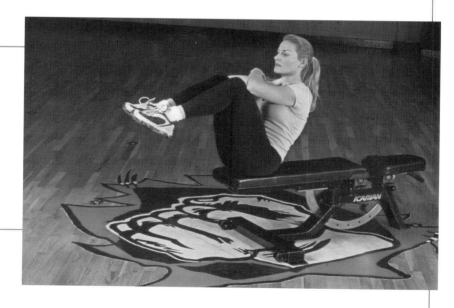

CARDIO WORKOUTS: DAYS 2, 4, AND 6

As in the Four-Week Workout, Days 2, 4, and 6 are cardio workouts—you can choose biking, jogging, brisk walking, swimming, etc. (We'll use jogging in our workout, but you can substitute your favorite activity.) Your cardio workouts will alternate between slow distance training in your fat-burning zone (three two-week periods) and cardio interval training (for three two-week periods).

You are exercising in your fat-burning zone when you are at 60 to 75% of your maximum heart rate (see the sidebar for how to calculate your maximum heart rate).

Here are the three stages of interval cardiovascular training:

1. Twenty-four minutes on cardiovascular equipment, rotating in six, two-minute intervals—for a total of six intervals of high intensity and six intervals of low intensity. For example, if you normally jog on the treadmill at a speed of 6.0, rotate in six, two-minute intervals sprinting at 8.0 for two minutes, then 6.0, then 8.0, etc. Today, you will have a shorter workout, but use 50% of your time at a high intensity.

2. Thirty-six minutes on the cardiovascular machine, again rotating six, two-minute intervals at a high intensity (e.g., four minutes at 6.0, then two minutes at 8.0, etc.). When you reach this step, you will operate at a 3:1 ratio of high intensity to your normal pace.

3. Forty-eight minutes on the cardiovascular machine, rotating six, two-minute intervals at a high intensity (e.g., six minutes at 6.0, then two minutes at 8.0).

CALCULATING YOUR MAXIMUM HEART RATE

Subtract your age from 220. Let's use a 20-year old as an example:

220 minus 20 years = 200 beats per minute (bpm)

200 bpm = maximum heart rate

60 to 75% intensity = 120 to 150 beats per minute

Heart rate monitors offer the most convenient readings, but a more practical approach is a six-second pulse count. Count the number of beats you feel in six seconds and multiply that by 10. For example, if our 20-year old counts 14 beats in six seconds, she is exercising at 140 beats per minute—well within her fat-burning zone.

WEEK 1

DAYS 1, 3, AND 5

Exercise	Reps / Time / Weight	
Warm up	5 minutes	
Stretch		
Jump rope	60 seconds	
Body squats	2 sets of 12	
ALT*: Stationary lunges	2 sets of 12 each leg	
Knee push-ups	2 sets of 12	
ALT: Exercise band rows	2 sets of 12	
Abs	3 sets	
Jump rope	60 seconds	
Step-ups	2 sets of 12	
Plié squats	2 sets of 12	
Dumbbell shoulder presses	2 sets of 12	5 lbs.
ALT: Dumbbell bicep curls	2 sets of 12	5 lbs.
ALT: Tricep kickbacks (extensions)	2 sets of 12	5 lbs.
Abdominal clams	3 sets of 20–25	
Jump rope	60 seconds	
Cool down/stretch		

*ALT: Alternate sets of the first exercise (preceding the one marked ALT) with sets of the next exercise (marked ALT).

DAYS 2, 4, AND 6

Begin slow distance training in your fat-burning zone:

   Day 2: Jog for 20 minutes
   Day 4: Jog for 22 minutes
   Day 6: Jog for 24 minutes

WEEK 2

DAYS 1, 3, AND 5

Exercise	Reps / Time / Weight	
Warm up	5 minutes	
Stretch		
Jump rope	90 seconds	
Body squats	2 sets of 12	5 lbs.
ALT: Stationary lunges	2 sets of 12	5 lbs.
Push-ups (regular)	2 sets of 4	
Push-ups (knees)	2 sets of 8	
ALT: Exercise band rows	2 sets of 12	
Abs	4 sets	
Jump rope	60 seconds	
Step-ups	2 sets of 12	5 lbs.
ALT: Plié squats	2 sets of 12	5 lbs.
Dumbbell shoulder presses	2 sets of 12	8 lbs.
ALT: Dumbbell bicep curls	2 sets of 12	8 lbs.
ALT: Tricep kickbacks	2 sets of 12	8 lbs.
Abdominal clams	3 sets of 20–25	
Jump rope	60 seconds	
Cool down/stretch		

DAYS 2, 4, AND 6

Continue slow distance training:

Day 2: Jog for 26 minutes
Day 4: Jog for 28 minutes
Day 6: Jog for 30 minutes

WEEK 3

DAYS 1, 3, AND 5

Exercise	Reps / Time / Weight	
Warm up/stretch		
Jump rope	90 seconds	
Body squats	2 sets of 12	8 lbs.
ALT: Stationary lunges	2 sets of 12	8 lbs.
Push-ups (regular)	2 sets of 8	
Push-ups (knees)	4	
ALT: Exercise band rows	2 sets of 12	
Abs	4 sets	
Jump rope	90 seconds	
Step-ups	2 sets of 12	8 lbs.
ALT: Plié squats	2 sets of 12	8 lbs.
Dumbbell shoulder presses	2 sets of 12	10 lbs.
ALT: Dumbbell bicep curls	2 sets of 12	10 lbs.
ALT: Bench dips	2 sets of 10	
ALT: Tricep kickbacks	2 sets of 12	
Abdominal clams	4 sets of 20–25	
Jump rope	60 seconds	
Cool down/stretch		

DAYS 2, 4, AND 6

Begin interval training by taking a 24-minute interval jog on each of the three days.

WEEK 4

DAYS 1, 3, 5

Exercise	Reps / Time / Weight	
Warm up/Stretch		
Jump rope	90 seconds	
Body squats	2 sets of 12	10 lbs.
ALT: Stationary lunges	2 sets of 12	10 lbs.
Push-ups (regular)	2 sets of 12	
ALT: Exercise band rows	2 sets of 12	
Abs	5 sets	
Jump rope	90 seconds	
Step-ups	2 sets of 12	10 lbs.
ALT: Plié squats	2 sets of 12	10 lbs.
Lateral raises	2 sets of 12	5 lbs.
ALT: Dumbbell shoulder presses	2 sets of 12	8 lbs.
ALT: Exercise band curls	2 sets of 12	
ALT: Dumbbell bicep curls	2 sets of 12	8 lbs.
ALT: Bench dips	2 sets of 12	
ALT: Tricep kickbacks	2 sets of 12	5 lbs.
Abdominal clams	4 sets of 25	
Jump rope	90 seconds	
Cool down/stretch		

DAYS 2, 4, AND 6

Continue interval training with the 24-minute interval jog on each of the three days.

WEEK 5

DAYS 1, 3, AND 5

Exercise	Reps / Time / Weight	
Warm up/Stretch		
Jump rope	2 minutes	
Body squats	2 sets of 12	10 lbs.
ALT: Squat thrusts	2 sets of 10	
ALT: Stationary lunges	2 sets of 12	10 lbs.
Pec flies	2 sets of 10	8 lbs.
ALT: Push-ups	2 sets of 12	
ALT: Rear delt raises	2 sets of 10	5 lbs.
ALT: Exercise band rows	2 sets of 12	
Abs	5 sets	
Jump rope	90 seconds	
Step-ups	2 sets of 12	10 lbs.
ALT: Mountain climbers	2 sets of 20	
ALT: Plié squats	2 sets of 12	10 lbs.
Lateral raises	2 sets of 12	5 lbs.
ALT: Dumbbell shoulder presses	2 sets of 12	10 lbs.
ALT: Exercise band curls	2 sets of 12	
ALT: Dumbbell bicep curls	2 sets of 12	10 lbs.
ALT: Bench dips	2 sets of 12	
ALT: Tricep kickbacks	2 sets of 12	8 lbs.
Abdominal clams	5 sets of 20	
Jump rope	90 seconds	
Cool down/stretch		

DAYS 2, 4, AND 6

Return to slow distance training:

Day 2: Jog for 30 minutes
Day 4: Jog for 32 minutes
Day 6: Jog for 34 minutes

WEEK 6

DAYS 1, 3, AND 5

Exercise	Reps / Time / Weight	
Warm up/Stretch		
Abs	2 sets of 20	
Jump rope	2 minutes	
Body squats	2 sets of 15	10 lbs.
ALT: Squat thrusts	2 sets of 10	
ALT: Stationary lunges	2 sets of 15	10 lbs.
Pec flies	2 sets of 10	8 lbs.
ALT: Push-ups	2 sets of 15	
ALT: Rear delt raises	2 sets of 10	5 lbs.
ALT: Exercise band rows	2 sets of 15	
Abs	5 sets of 20	
Jump rope	2 minutes	
Step-ups	2 sets of 15	10 lbs.
ALT: Mountain climbers	2 sets of 20	
ALT: Plié squats	2 sets of 15	10 lbs.
Lateral raises	2 sets of 12	5 lbs.
ALT: Dumbbell shoulder presses	2 sets of 15	10 lbs.
ALT: Exercise band curls	2 sets of 12	
ALT: Dumbbell bicep curls	2 sets of 15	10 lbs.
ALT: Bench dips	2 sets of 12	
ALT: Tricep kickbacks	2 sets of 15	8 lbs.
Abdominal clams	5 sets of 20	
Jump rope	90 seconds	
Cool down/stretch		

DAYS 2, 4, AND 6

Continue slow distance training:

Day 2: Jog for 36 minutes
Day 4: Jog for 38 minutes
Day 6: Jog for 40 minutes

WEEK 7

DAYS 1, 3, AND 5

Exercise	Reps / Time / Weight	
Warm up/Stretch		
Abs	3 sets of 20	
Jump rope	2 minutes	
Body squats	2 sets of 15	10 lbs.
ALT: Squat thrusts	2 sets of 15	
ALT: Stationary lunges	2 sets of 15	10 lbs.
Pec flies	2 sets of 15	8 lbs.
ALT: Push-ups	2 sets of 15	
ALT: Rear delt raises	2 sets of 15	5 lbs.
ALT: Exercise band rows	2 sets of 15	
Abs	5 sets of 20	
Jump rope	2 minutes	
Step-ups	2 sets of 15	10 lbs.
ALT: Mountain climbers	2 sets of 25	
ALT: Plié squats	2 sets of 15	10 lbs.
Lateral raises	2 sets of 15	5 lbs.
ALT: Dumbbell shoulder presses	2 sets of 15	10 lbs.
ALT: Exercise band curls	2 sets of 15	
ALT: Dumbbell bicep curls	2 sets of 15	10 lbs.
ALT: Bench dips	2 sets of 15	
ALT: Tricep kickbacks	2 sets of 15	8 lbs.
Abdominal clams	5 sets of 20	
Jump rope	90 seconds	
Cool down/stretch		

DAYS 2, 4, AND 6

Resume interval training with the 36-minute interval jog on each of the three days.

WEEK 8

DAYS 1, 3, AND 5

Exercise	Reps / Time / Weight	
Warmup/Stretch		
Abs	4 sets of 20	
Jump rope	2 minutes	
Jumping jacks	25	
Body squats	3 sets of 15	10 lbs.
ALT: Squat thrusts	3 sets of 15	
ALT: Stationary lunges	3 sets of 15	10 lbs.
Pec flies	3 sets of 15	8 lbs.
ALT: Push-ups	3 sets of 15	
ALT: Rear delt raises	3 sets of 15	5 lbs.
ALT: Exercise band rows	3 sets of 15	
Body squats	1 set of 15	10 lbs.
ALT: Push-ups	1 set of 15	
Abs	5 sets of 20	
Jump rope	2 minutes	
Step-ups	3 sets of 15	10 lbs.
ALT: Mountain climbers	3 sets of 30	
ALT: Plié squats	3 sets of 15	10 lbs.
Lateral raises	3 sets of 15	5 lbs.
ALT: Dumbbell shoulder presses	3 sets of 15	10 lbs.
ALT: Exercise band curls	3 sets of 15	
ALT: Dumbbell bicep curls	3 sets of 15	10 lbs.
ALT: Bench dips	3 sets of 15	
ALT: Tricep kickbacks	3 sets of 15	8 lbs.
Abdominal clams	5 sets of 20	
Jump rope	2 minutes	
Cool down/stretch		

DAYS 2, 4, AND 6

Continue interval training with the 36-minute interval jog on each of the three days.

WEEK 9

DAYS 1, 3, AND 5

Exercise	Reps / Time / Weight	
Warm up/Stretch		
Abs	4 sets of 20	
Jump rope	2 minutes	
Jumping jacks	25	
Body squats	3 sets of 15	10 lbs.
ALT: Squat thrusts	3 sets of 15	
ALT: Stationary lunges	3 sets of 15	10 lbs.
Pec flies	3 sets of 15	8 lbs.
ALT: Push-ups	3 sets of 15	
ALT: Rear delt raises	3 sets of 15	5 lbs.
ALT: Exercise band rows	3 sets of 15	
Body squats	1 set of 15	10 lbs.
ALT: Push-ups	1 set of 15	
Abs	5 sets of 20	
Jump rope	2 minutes	
Jumping jacks	25	
Step-ups	3 sets of 15	10 lbs.
ALT: Mountain climbers	3 sets of 30	
ALT: Plié squats	3 sets of 15	10 lbs.
Lateral raises	3 sets of 15	5 lbs.
ALT: Dumbbell shoulder presses	3 sets of 15	10 lbs.
ALT: Exercise band curls	3 sets of 15	
ALT: Dumbbell bicep curls	3 sets of 15	10 lbs.
ALT: Bench dips	3 sets of 15	
ALT: Tricep kickbacks	3 sets of 15	8 lbs.
Shoulder presses	1 set of 15	10 lbs.
ALT: Step-ups	1 set of 15	10 lbs.
Abs	5 sets of 20	
Jump rope	90 seconds	
Cool down/stretch		

DAYS 2, 4, AND 6

Resume slow distance training:

Day 2: Jog for 40 minutes
Day 4: Jog for 42 minutes
Day 6: Jog for 44 minutes

WEEK 10

DAYS 1, 3, AND 5

Exercise	Reps / Time / Weight	
Warm up/Stretch		
Abs	5 sets of 20	
Jump rope	2 minutes	
Jumping Jacks	25	
Body squats	3 sets of 15	10 lbs.
ALT: Squat thrusts	3 sets of 15	
ALT: Stationary lunges	3 sets of 15	10 lbs.
Pec flies	3 sets of 15	8 lbs.
ALT: Push-ups	3 sets of 15	
ALT: Rear delt raises	3 sets of 15	5 lbs.
ALT: Exercise band rows	3 sets of 15	
Body squats	1 set of 15	10 lbs.
ALT: Push-ups	1 set of 15	
ALT: Stationary lunges	1 set of 15	10 lbs.
ALT: Exercise band rows	1 set of 15	
Abs	5 sets of 20	
Jump rope	2 minutes	
Jumping jacks	25	
Step-ups	3 sets of 15	10 lbs.
ALT: Mountain climbers	3 sets of 30	
ALT: Plié squats	3 sets of 15	10 lbs.
Lateral raises	3 sets of 15	5 lbs.
ALT: Dumbbell shoulder presses	3 sets of 15	10 lbs.
ALT: Exercise band curls	3 sets of 15	
ALT: Dumbbell bicep curls	3 sets of 15	10 lbs.
ALT: Bench dips	3 sets of 15	
ALT: Tricep kickbacks	3 sets of 15	8 lbs.
Shoulder presses	1 set of 15	10 lbs.
ALT: Step-ups	1 set of 15	10 lbs.
ALT: Bicep curls	1 set of 15	10 lbs.
Abs	5 sets of 20	
Jump rope	90 seconds	
Jumping jacks	25	
Cool down/stretch		

DAYS 2, 4, AND 6

Continue slow distance training:

Day 2: Jog for 46 minutes
Day 4: Jog for 48 minutes
Day 6: Jog for 50 minutes

WEEK 11

DAYS 1, 3, AND 5

Exercise	Reps / Time / Weight	
Warm up/Stretch		
Abs	5 sets of 20	
Jump rope	2 minutes	
Jumping jacks	25	
Body squats	3 sets of 15	10 lbs.
ALT: Squat thrusts	3 sets of 15	
ALT: Stationary lunges	3 sets of 15	10 lbs.
Pec flies	3 sets of 15	8 lbs.
ALT: Push-ups	3 sets of 15	
ALT: Rear delt raises	3 sets of 15	5 lbs.
ALT: Exercise band rows	3 sets of 15	
Body squats	2 sets of 15	10 lbs.
ALT: Push-ups	2 sets of 15	
ALT: Stationary lunges	1 set of 15	10 lbs.
ALT: Exercise band rows	1 set of 15	
Abs	5 sets of 20	
Jump rope	2 minutes	
Jumping jacks	25	
Step-ups	3 sets of 15	10 lbs.
ALT: Mountain climbers	3 sets of 30	
ALT: Plié squats	3 sets of 15	10 lbs.
Lateral raises	3 sets of 15	5 lbs.
ALT: Dumbbell shoulder presses	3 sets of 15	10 lbs.
ALT: Exercise band curls	3 sets of 15	
ALT: Dumbbell bicep curls	3 sets of 15	10 lbs.
ALT: Bench dips	3 sets of 15	
ALT: Tricep kickbacks	3 sets of 15	8 lbs.
Shoulder presses	1 set of 15	10 lbs.
ALT: Step-ups	1 set of 15	10 lbs.
ALT: Bicep curls	1 set of 15	10 lbs.
Abs	5 sets of 20	
Jump rope	90 seconds	
Jumping jacks	25	
Cool down/stretch		

DAYS 2, 4, AND 6

Resume interval training with the 48-minute interval jog on each of the three days.

WEEK 12

DAYS 1, 3, AND 5

Exercise	Reps / Time / Weight	
Warm up/Stretch		
Abs	5 sets of 20	
Jump rope	2 minutes	
Jumping jacks	25	
Body squats	3 sets of 15	10 lbs.
ALT: Squat thrusts	3 sets of 15	
ALT: Stationary lunges	3 sets of 15	10 lbs.
Pec flies	3 sets of 15	8 lbs.
ALT: Push-ups	3 sets of 15	
ALT: Rear delt raises	3 sets of 15	5 lbs.
ALT: Exercise band rows	3 sets of 15	
Body squats	2 sets of 15	10 lbs.
ALT: Push-ups	2 sets of 15	
ALT: Stationary lunges	2 sets of 15	10 lbs.
ALT: Exercise band rows	2 sets of 15	
Abs	5 sets of 20	
Jump rope	2 minutes	
Jumping jacks	25	
Step-ups	3 sets of 15	10 lbs.
ALT: Mountain climbers	3 sets of 30	
ALT: Plié squats	3 sets of 15	10 lbs.
Lateral raises	3 sets of 15	5 lbs.
ALT: Dumbbell shoulder presses	3 sets of 15	10 lbs.
ALT: Exercise band curls	3 sets of 15	
ALT: Dumbbell bicep curls	3 sets of 15	10 lbs.
ALT: Bench dips	3 sets of 15	
ALT: Tricep kickbacks	3 sets of 15	8 lbs.
Shoulder presses	2 sets of 15	10 lbs.
ALT: Step-ups	2 sets of 15	10 lbs.
ALT: Bicep curls	2 sets of 15	10 lbs.
Abs	5 sets of 20	
Jump rope	2 minutes	
Jumping jacks	25	
Cool down/stretch		

DAYS 2, 4 AND 6

Continue interval training with the 48-minute interval jog of the three days each hand.

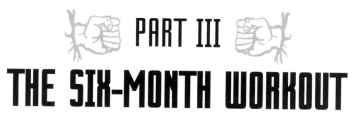

PART III
THE SIX-MONTH WORKOUT

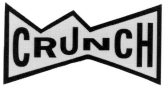

You're planning ahead for the big day, and CRUNCH is going to make sure you reach your goal with the Six-Month Workout.

STRENGTH TRAINING

As in the Four-Week and 12-Week Workouts, the Six-Month Workout alternates days of cardio workouts with days of strength training workouts.

Days 1, 3, and 5 of each week are strength training days. Allow an hour for your workouts on these days. Each workout includes all the major muscle groups. Try not to take much time between sets.

The six-month strength-training program is designed to use free weights not only to condition and tone your muscles but to burn fat as the energy source throughout the workout. The two minutes on the treadmill following the warm-up and stretch should actually raise the heart rate above your fat-burning target heart rate.

Your fat-burning heart rate is 65 to 75% of your maximum heart rate (see sidebar for calculating your maximum heart rate). Once you reach 75 to 80% of your maximum heart rate—known as the "anaerobic threshold"—you are actually past your fat-burning zone. Why cross that anaerobic threshold if you're not burning fat? By pushing yourself past that threshold, the threshold will eventually get higher and higher, which means that your fat-burning zone, or "aerobic capacity," will increase.

The first round of leg exercises will keep your heart rate in the middle to upper half of the fat-burning target zone. As you complete the pecs and back exercises, your heart rate will be toward the very

CALCULATING YOUR MAXIMUM HEART RATE

Subtract your age from 220. Let's use a 20-year old as an example:

220 minus 20 years = 200 beats per minute (bpm)

200 bpm = maximum heart rate

65 to 75% intensity = 120 to 150 beats per minute

Heart rate monitors offer the most convenient readings, but a more practical approach is a six-second pulse count. Count the number of beats you feel in six seconds and multiply that by 10. For example, if our 20-year old counts 14 beats in six seconds, she is exercising at 140 beats per minute—well within her fat-burning zone.

bottom of the fat-burning zone. At that point two minutes on the stationary bike will elevate the heart rate again, above the anaerobic threshold.

The second half of the workout will begin with an additional round of leg exercises followed by completion of the upper body workout in a shoulder, bicep, and tricep sequence. The workout winds up with abdominal and lower back conditioning.

Weeks 1 through 3 use basic movements using both free weights and machine exercises. A strong base for the weeks to come is established.

In Weeks 4 through 12, the intensity of the program is increased. Weight is added to half of the leg exercises in both the first and second parts of the lower body routine, as well as the chest/back and shoulder/bicep/tricep sequences. Weight is increased in a few exercises at a time so the increase in difficulty is gradual.

In Week 13, the leg press is added to the first round of leg exercises and the dumbbell and plie squats are moved to the second round of leg exercises. Both rounds will be more challenging. The back and chest workload is increased by adding cable rows and pec flies to the mix. Lateral raises, cable curls, and bench dips are added to challenge the shoulders, biceps, and triceps, respectively.

In Week 13, the cardio intervals (two minutes on treadmill and bike) change as well. The two minutes are broken down into 30 seconds of moderate intensity followed by 30 seconds of high intensity. Repeating this cycle will increase your aerobic capacity.

In Week 19, reps are lowered and weight is added to increase muscle density. At this point, tougher abdominal exercises are added to keep pace with the tougher workouts for the other muscle groups. Side bends are added to tighten obliques.

In Week 25, the workout switches to a "pre-exhaust mode." Secondary exercises, such as the pec fly after the dumbbell chest press, are reversed. Doing the pec fly first increases the difficulty of the dumbbell chest press without having to add weight or reps. This principle is applied to both rounds of leg exercises and to the entire upper body as well.

Before we lay out the weekly program for the Six-Month Workout, let's review how to do each exercise correctly.

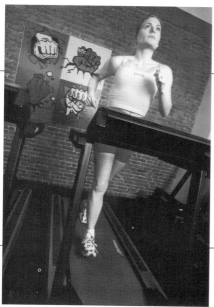 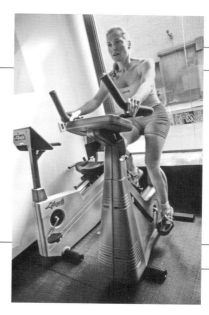

WARM UP AND STRETCH:

You should warm up with five minutes of light cardio activity on each day. You don't want to push yourself—you just want to warm your muscles before you stretch them out. Doing so produces synovial fluid, which is a lubricant for your joints and helps prevent injury. After your warm-up, make sure your stretch involves all the major muscle groups.

DUMBBELL SQUATS:

This is an excellent exercise that targets the hamstrings. Place your feet shoulder-width apart and hold dumbbells in each hand. Lower your body toward the floor until your thighs are parallel to the floor and then return to a standing position.

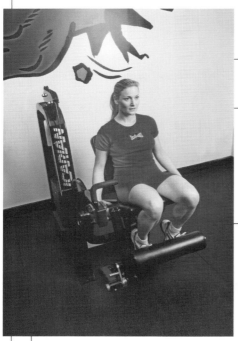

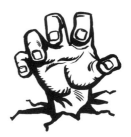

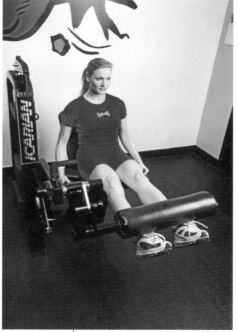

LEG EXTENSION (QUAD-RICEPS):

While sitting, holding the bars at your sides, and resting the pad on top of your ankles, slowly raise the pad till your legs are fully extended in front of you (don't lock your knees). The bottom point of the movement should be near straight leg. Raise pad behind heels up to a right angle between upper and lower leg.

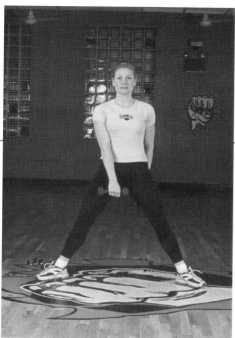

PLIÉ SQUATS:

For these squats, your feet should be
pointed slightly outward. Bend your
knees out to the sides as you squat.
You can stretch your arms out to the
side for balance.

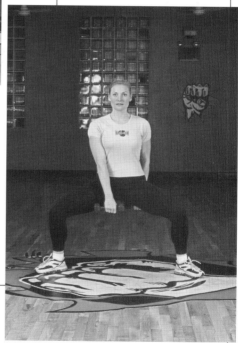

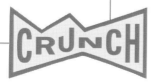

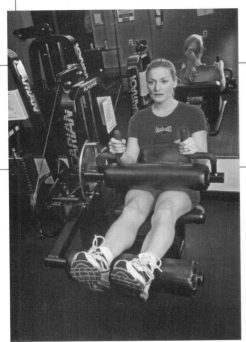

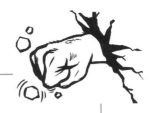

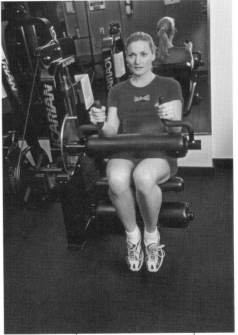

LEG CURLS
(HAMSTRINGS, GLUTES):

Sitting and grabbing the bars with both hands, lower weight slowly down to a bottom point of a right angle between the upper leg and lower leg. Flex at the knee, raising the feet until almost completely straight-legged.

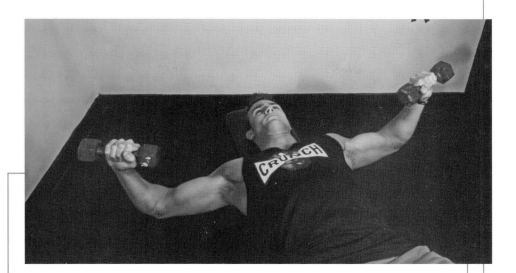

DUMBBELL CHEST PRESS (PECS):

Lie flat on the bench, pinching shoulder blades together to minimize shoulder effort. Lower dumbbells from near straight arm (do not lock elbows) down to just below right angle between forearm and upper arm, and raise them up again.

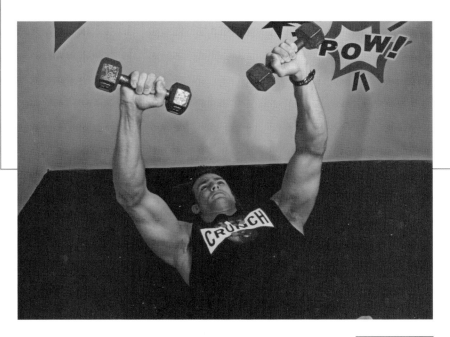

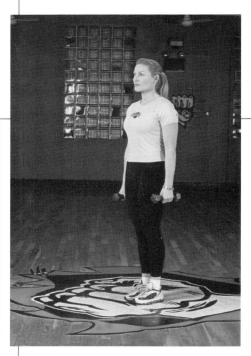

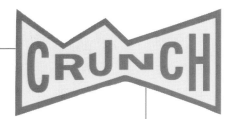

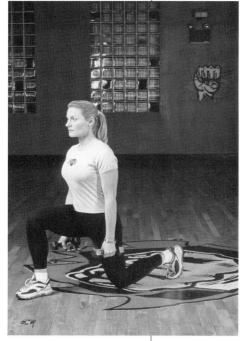

STATIONARY LUNGES:

Standing with legs shoulder-width apart and knees soft, take a step approximately 1.5 times your normal stride forward. Raise the heel of the back leg up so that you're standing on the balls of your foot. From this position, keeping the upper body over the torso, bend the back leg, bringing its knee to the ground. Raise up and repeat.

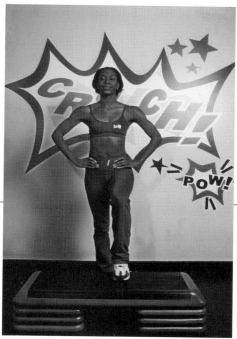

STEP-UPS:

These are done on steps or stairs or with a flat bench surface. The step should be no higher than your hips. One foot should be elevated on the step, while the second foot stays flat on the floor. After a slight push off from the lower leg, the top leg extends from a near right angle (shin and thigh) to an almost straight leg. **Trainer tip:** Don't lock your knee!

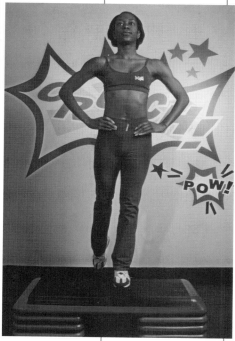

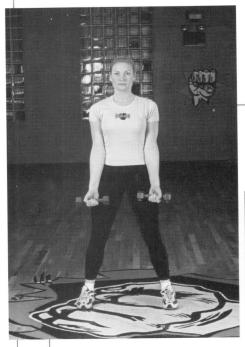

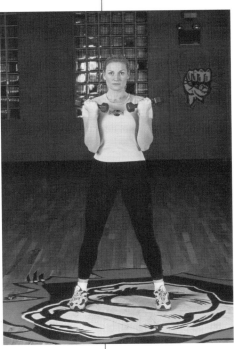

DUMBBELL BICEP CURLS:

Put your elbows at your sides and face your palms up. Lower the dumbbell toward the floor and then curl the dumbbell up to your shoulders.

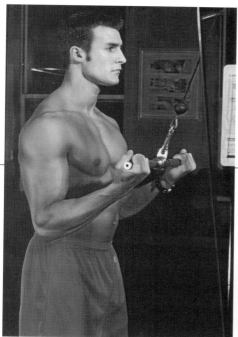

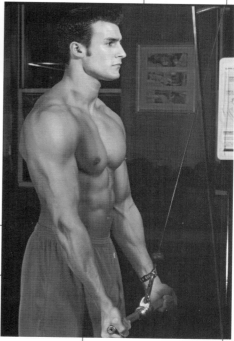

STRAIGHT BAR CABLE PULLDOWN (LATS):

Grip the bar just outside shoulder width apart. Pull the bar down to your legs till your arms are nearly straight.

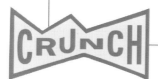

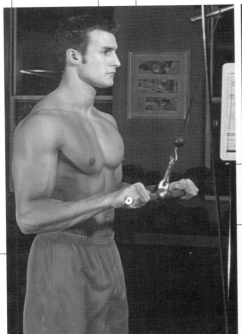 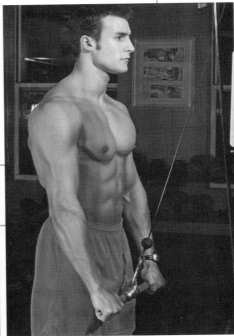

CABLE PUSHDOWN (TRICEPS):

Bend your knees slightly and pinch in your elbows. Push the handles down from a top point of just above a right angle between upper and lower arm to a bottom point of a near completely straightened arm.

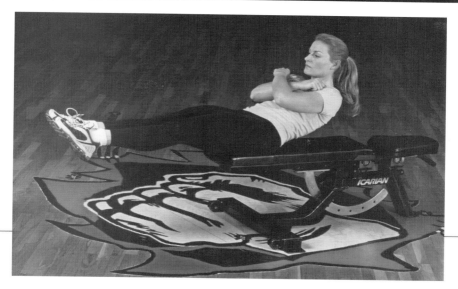

ABDOMINAL EXERCISES:

Abdominal clams are an excellent ab exercise because they recruit both lower and upper abdominal regions. Begin with your hands behind your neck (or across your chest) and keep your bent knees and feet elevated. Curl the upper body up and draw the knees into the body at the same time. **Trainer tip**: Be sure to avoid pulling in the neck!

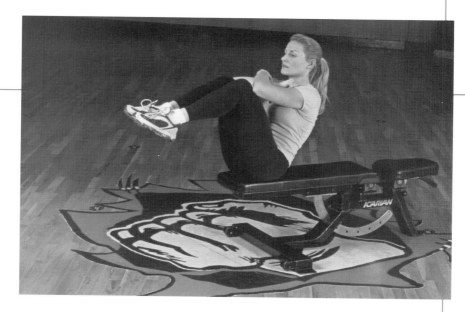

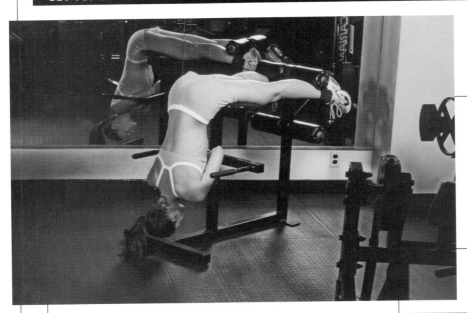

LOWER BACK EXTENSIONS:

Begin with pad at waist level. Lower your torso to form a right angle between your legs and upper body. Return to complete upright position.

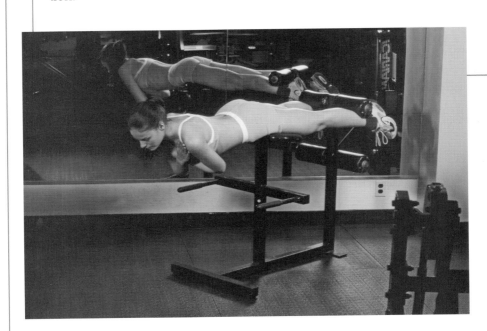

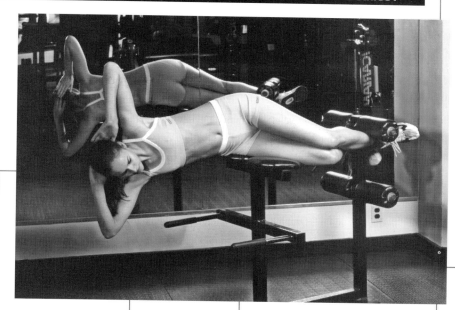

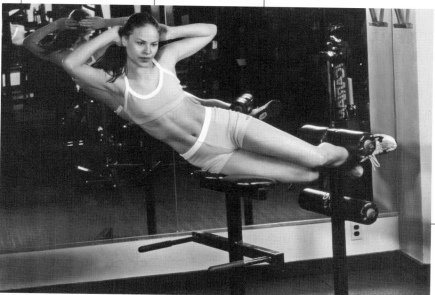

SIDE BENDS:

Begin on your side with the pad at hip level. Put your hands back behind your head and your elbows out to the side. Lean out and down with front elbow and return up and back with rear elbow.

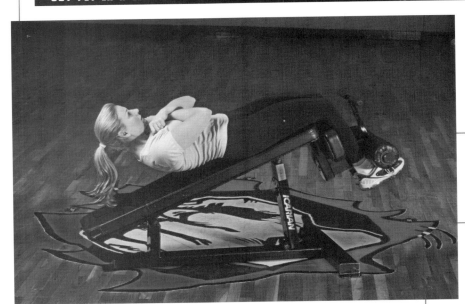

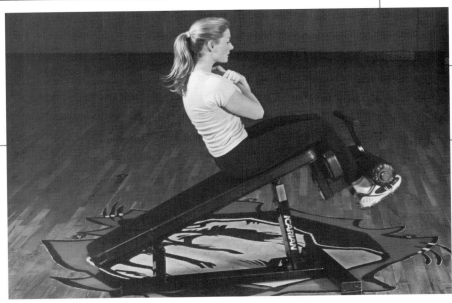

DECLINE CRUNCHES:

To increase difficulty of abdominal crunches, do them on a decline bench.

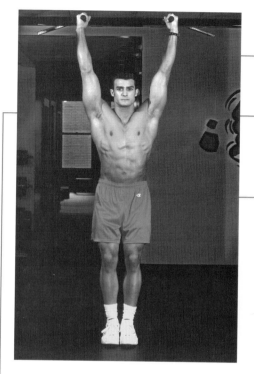

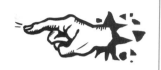

HANGING RAISES:

Hanging from a pull-up bar or pegs, contract abdominals so that knees are brought to waist level with feet extended out. Keep feet together and separate knees to minimize effort from the hip flexor muscles.

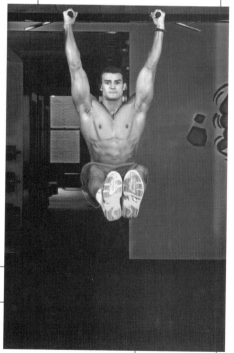

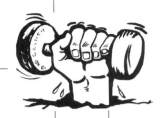

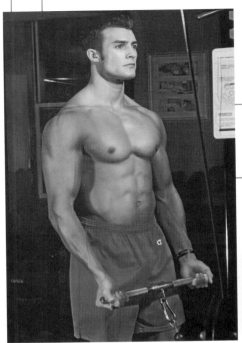

CABLE CURLS:

Stand with feet shoulder-width apart and hips square, facing weight stack. Using straight cable bar, move from a position of a nearly straight arm up 75 percent of the way to the shoulder. Keep elbows stationary, in tight to the rib cage.

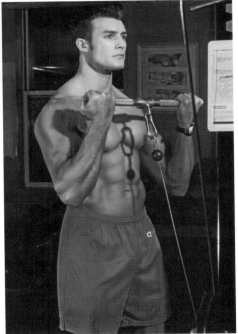

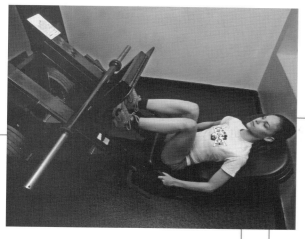

LEG PRESS:

Feet may be high or low on the platform, shoulder-width apart. Press the weights up until your legs are nearly straight (do not lock knees). With feet low on the platform, the exercise will recruit more effort from the quadriceps. With feet high on the platform, the exercise will recruit more effort from hamstrings and glutes.

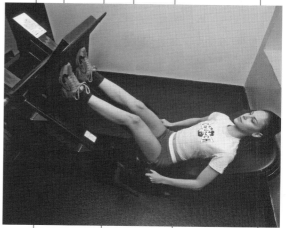

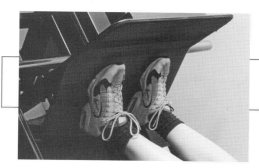

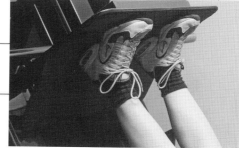

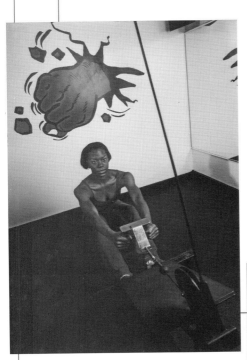

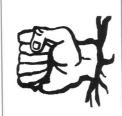

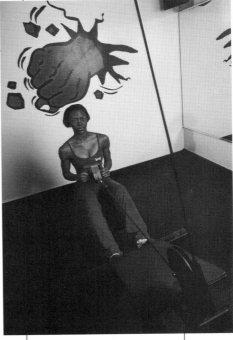

CABLE ROWS:

Your feet should be on the platform. Your legs should be almost straight, but with a slight bend in your knees. Keep your back straight. Begin with your arms completely extended forward. Retract your shoulder blades together, then flex your elbows so that your hands bring the handle in just below chest level. Keep your elbows in tight to your body.

CARDIO WORKOUTS: DAYS 2, 4, AND 6

Days 2, 4, and 6 of each week are cardio workouts—you can choose biking, jogging, brisk walking, swimming, etc. (We'll use jogging in the workout below, but you can substitute an alternate activity.) Your cardio workout will alternate in three-week cycles: three weeks of slow distance training in your fat-burning zone and three weeks of interval training.

Here are the three stages of interval cardiovascular training:

1. Twenty-four minutes on cardiovascular equipment, rotating in six, two-minute intervals—for a total of six intervals of high intensity and six intervals of low intensity. For example, if you normally jog on the treadmill at a speed of 6.0, rotate in six, two-minute intervals sprinting at 8.0 for two minutes, then 6.0, then 8.0, etc. Today, you will have a shorter workout, but use 50% of your time at a high intensity.

2. Thirty-six minutes on the cardiovascular machine, again rotating six, two-minute intervals at a high intensity (e.g., four minutes at 6.0, then two minutes at 8.0, etc.). When you reach this step, you will operate at a 3:1 ratio of high intensity to your normal pace.

3. Forty-eight minutes on the cardiovascular machine, rotating six, two-minute intervals at a high intensity (e.g., six minutes at 6.0, then two minutes at 8.0).

WEEKS 1-3

DAYS 1, 3, 5

Exercise	Reps / Time / Weight	
Warm up/Stretch		
Treadmill	2 minutes	
(heart rate above aerobic training zone)		
Dumbbell squats	1 set of 12	5 lbs.
Leg extensions	1 set of 12	10 lbs.
Plié squats	1 set of 12	5 lbs.
Leg curls	1 set of 12	10 lbs.
Dumbbell chest presses	1 set of 12	5 lbs.
Straight bar cable pulldowns	1 set of 12	40 lbs.
Stationary bike	2 minutes	
(heart rate above aerobic training zone)		
Step-ups	1 set of 12	5 lbs.
Stationary lunges	1 set of 12 per leg	5 lbs.
Step-ups	1 set of 12 per leg	5 lbs.
Dumbbell shoulder presses	1 set of 12	5 lbs.
Dumbbell bicep curls	1 set of 12	5 lbs.
Cable pushdowns	1 set of 12	25 lbs.
Dumbbell shoulder presses	1 set of 12	5 lbs.
Dumbbell bicep curls	1 set of 12	5 lbs.
Tricep cable pushdowns	1 set of 12	25 lbs.
Abdominal exercises	3 sets of 20	
(25 second rest between sets)		
Lower back extensions	1 set	
Stretch		

DAYS 2, 4, 6

In Week 1, begin slow distance training by jogging for 20 minutes on each of the three days. In Week 2, jog for 25 minutes on each of the three days. In Week 3, jog for 30 minutes on each of the cardio days.

WEEKS 4-6

DAYS 1, 3, AND 5

Exercise	Reps / Time / Weight	
Warm up/Stretch		
Treadmill	2 minutes	
(heart rate above aerobic training zone)		
Dumbbell squats	1 set of 12	8 lbs.
Leg extensions	1 set of 12	10 lbs.
Plié squats	1 set of 12	8 lbs.
Leg curls	1 set of 12	10 lbs.
Dumbbell chest presses	1 set of 12	8 lbs.
Straight bar cable pulldowns	1 set of 12	45 lbs.
Dumbbell chest presses	1 set of 12	5 lbs.
Straight bar cable pulldowns	1 set of 12	40 lbs.
Stationary bike	2 minutes	
(heart rate above aerobic training zone)		
Step-ups	1 set of 12	8 lbs.
Stationary lunges	1 set of 12 per leg	8 lbs.
Step-ups	1 set of 12 per leg	5 lbs.
Stationary lunges	1 set of 12 per leg	5 lbs.
Dumbbell shoulder presses	1 set of 12	8 lbs.
Dumbbell bicep curls	1 set of 12	8 lbs.
Cable pushdowns	1 set of 12	30 lbs.
Dumbbell shoulder presses	1 set of 12	5 lbs.
Dumbbell bicep curls	1 set of 12	5 lbs.
Tricep cable pushdowns	1 set of 12	25 lbs.
Abdominal exercises	4 sets of 20	
(25 second rest between sets)		
Lower back extensions	2 sets	
Stretch		

DAYS 2, 4, 6

Begin interval training by going for a 24-minute interval jog on each of the three days for all three weeks.

WEEKS 7-9

DAYS 1, 3, AND 5

Exercise	Reps / Time / Weight	
Warm up/Stretch		
Treadmill	2 minutes	
(heart rate above aerobic training zone)		
Dumbbell squats	1 set of 12	8 lbs.
Leg extensions	1 set of 12	20 lbs.
Plié squats	1 set of 12	8 lbs.
Leg curls	1 set of 12	30 lbs.
Dumbbell chest presses	1 set of 12	8 lbs.
Straight bar cable pulldowns	1 set of 12	45 lbs.
Dumbbell chest presses	1 set of 12	8 lbs.
Straight bar cable pulldowns	1 set of 12	45 lbs.
Stationary bike	2 minutes	
(heart rate above aerobic training zone)		
Step-ups	1 set of 12	8 lbs.
Stationary lunges	1 set of 12 per leg	8 lbs.
Step-ups	1 set of 12 per leg	8 lbs.
Stationary lunges	1 set of 12 per leg	8 lbs.
Dumbbell shoulder presses	1 set of 12	8 lbs.
Dumbbell bicep curls	1 set of 12	8 lbs.
Cable pushdowns	1 set of 12	30 lbs.
Dumbbell shoulder presses	1 set of 12	8 lbs.
Dumbbell bicep curls	1 set of 12	8 lbs.
Tricep cable pushdowns	1 set of 12	30 lbs.
Abdominal exercises	5 sets of 20	
(25 second rest between sets)		
Lower back extensions	2 sets	
Stretch		

DAYS 2, 4, 6

In Week 7, resume slow distance training by jogging for 30 minutes on each of the three days. In Week 8, jog for 35 minutes on each of the three days. In Week 9, jog for 40 minutes on each of the cardio days.

WEEKS 10-12

DAYS 1, 3, AND 5

Exercise	Reps / Time / Weight	
Warm up/Stretch		
Treadmill	2 minutes	
(heart rate above aerobic training zone)		
Dumbbell squats	1 set of 12	10 lbs.
Leg extensions	1 set of 12	30 lbs.
Plié squats	1 set of 12	10 lbs.
Leg curls	1 set of 12	30 lbs.
Dumbbell chest presses	1 set of 12	10 lbs.
Straight bar cable pulldowns	1 set of 12	50 lbs.
Dumbbell chest presses	1 set of 12	10 lbs.
Straight bar cable pulldowns	1 set of 12	50 lbs.
Stationary bike	2 minutes	
(heart rate above aerobic training zone)		
Step-ups	1 set of 12	10 lbs.
Stationary lunges	1 set of 12 per leg	10 lbs.
Step-ups	1 set of 12 per leg	10 lbs.
Stationary lunges	1 set of 12 per leg	10 lbs.
Dumbbell shoulder presses	1 set of 12	10 lbs.
Dumbbell bicep curls	1 set of 12	10 lbs.
Cable pushdowns	1 set of 12	35 lbs.
Dumbbell shoulder presses	1 set of 12	10 lbs.
Dumbbell bicep curls	1 set of 12	10 lbs.
Tricep cable pushdowns	1 set of 12	35 lbs.
Abdominal exercises	6 sets of 20	
(25 second rest between sets)		
Lower back extensions	3 sets	
Stretch		

DAYS 2, 4, 6

Resume interval training by going for a 36-minute interval jog on each of the three days for all three weeks.

WEEKS 13-15

DAYS 1, 3, AND 5

Exercise	Reps / Time / Weight	
Warm up/Stretch		
Treadmill	30 sec. walk / 30 second jog	
Treadmill	30 sec. walk / 30 second jog	
Leg presses (feet low)	1 set of 12	20 lbs.
Leg extensions	1 set of 12	30 lbs.
Leg presses (feet high)	1 set of 12	20 lbs.
Leg curls	1 set of 12	30 lbs.
Dumbbell chest presses	1 set of 12	10 lbs.
Dumbbell pec flies	1 set of 12	8 lbs.
Straight-bar cable pulldowns	1 set of 12	50 lbs.
Cable rows	1 set of 12	35 lbs.
Dumbbell chest presses	1 set of 12	10 lbs.
Straight-bar cable pulldowns	1 set of 12	50 lbs.
Stationary bike	30 sec. mod. intensity/30 sec. high intensity	
Stationary bike	30 sec. mod. intensity/30 sec. high intensity	
Dumbbell squats	1 set of 12	10 lbs.
Step-ups	1 set of 12	10 lbs.
Plié squats	1 set of 12	10 lbs.
Stationary lunges	1 set of 12 per leg	10 lbs.
Lateral raises	1 set of 12	5 lbs.
Dumbbell bicep curls	1 set of 12	10 lbs.
Cable bicep curls	1 set of 12	25 lbs.
Tricep cable pushdowns	1 set of 12	35 lbs.
Bench dips	1 set of 12	
Dumbbell shoulder presses	1 set of 12	10 lbs.
Dumbbell bicep curls	1 set of 12	10 lbs.
Tricep cable pushdowns	1 set of 12	35 lbs.
Decline crunches	1 set of 20	
Abs (on floor)	5 sets of 20	
Side bends	1 set of 20 per side	
Lower back extensions	3 sets of 20	
Stretch		

DAYS 2, 4, 6

In Week 13, resume slow distance training by jogging for 40 minutes on each of the three days. In Week 14, jog for 45 minutes on each of the three days. In Week 15, jog for 50 minutes on each of the cardio days.

WEEKS 16-18

DAYS 1, 3, AND 5

Exercise	Reps / Time / Weight	
Warm up/Stretch		
Treadmill	30 sec. walk / 30 second jog	
Leg presses (feet low)	1 set of 12	35 lbs.
Leg extensions	1 set of 12	30 lbs.
Leg presses (feet high)	1 set of 12	30 lbs.
Leg curls	1 set of 12	30 lbs.
Dumbbell chest presses	1 set of 12	10 lbs.
Dumbbell pec flies	1 set of 12	8 lbs.
Straight-bar cable pulldowns	1 set of 12	50 lbs.
Cable rows	1 set of 12	35 lbs.
Dumbbell pec flies	1 set of 12	8 lbs.
Straight-bar cable pulldowns	1 set of 12	50 lbs.
Cable rows	1 set of 12	35 lbs.
Stationary bike	30 sec. mod. intensity/30 sec. high intensity	
Dumbbell squats	1 set of 12	10 lbs.
Step-ups	1 set of 12	10 lbs.
Plié squats	1 set of 12	10 lbs.
Stationary lunges	1 set of 12 per leg	10 lbs.
Dumbbell squats	1 set of 12	10 lbs.
Step-ups	1 set of 12	10 lbs.
Dumbbell shoulder presses	1 set of 10	12 lbs.
Lateral raises	1 set of 12	5 lbs.
Dumbbell bicep curls	1 set of 12	12 lbs.
Cable bicep curls	1 set of 10	25 lbs.
Tricep cable pushdowns	1 set of 12	40 lbs.
Bench dips	1 set of 12	
Dumbbell shoulder presses	1 set of 10	12 lbs.
Lateral raises	1 set of 12	5 lbs.
Dumbbell bicep curls	1 set of 12	12 lbs.
Cable bicep curls	1 set of 12	25 lbs.
Tricep cable pushdowns	1 set of 10	40 lbs.
Bench dips	1 set of 12	
Hanging leg raises	1 set of 20	
Decline crunches	1 set of 20	
Abs (on floor)	3 sets of 20	
Side bends	3 sets of 20 per side	
Lower back extensions	3 sets of 20	
Stretch		

DAYS 2, 4, 6 [WEEKS 16-18 CONTINUED]

Resume interval training by going for a 48-minute interval jog on each of the three days for all three weeks.

WEEKS 19 - 21

DAYS 1, 3, AND 5

Exercise	Reps / Time / Weight	
Warm up/Stretch		
Treadmill	2 minutes high intensity	
Leg presses (feet low)	1 set of 12	50 lbs.
Leg extensions	1 set of 12	30 lbs.
Leg extensions	1 set of 12	10 lbs.
Leg presses (feet high)	1 set of 12	50 lbs.
Leg curls	1 set of 12	30 lbs.
Leg curls	1 set of 12	10 lbs.
Dumbbell chest presses	1 set of 10	12 lbs.
Dumbbell pec flies	1 set of 10	10 lbs.
Straight-bar cable pulldowns	1 set of 10	60 lbs.
Cable rows	1 set of 10	40 lbs.
Dumbbell chest presses	1 set of 10	12 lbs.
Dumbbell pec flies	1 set of 10	8 lbs.
Straight-bar cable pulldowns	1 set of 10	50 lbs.
Cable rows	1 set of 10	40 lbs.
Stationary bike	2 minutes high intensity	
Dumbbell shoulder presses	1 set of 10	12 lbs.
Lateral raises	1 set of 12	5 lbs.
Dumbbell bicep curls	1 set of 12	12 lbs.
Cable bicep curls	1 set of 10	25 lbs.
Tricep cable pushdowns	1 set of 12	40 lbs.
Bench dips	1 set of 12	
Dumbbell shoulder presses	1 set of 10	12 lbs.
Lateral raises	1 set of 12	5 lbs.
Dumbbell bicep curls	1 set of 12	12 lbs.
Cable bicep curls	1 set of 12	25 lbs.
Tricep cable pushdowns	1 set of 10	40 lbs.
Bench dips	1 set of 12	
Hanging leg raises	1 set of 20	
Decline crunches	2 sets of 20	
Abs (on floor)	3 sets of 20	
Side bends	3 sets of 20 per side	
Lower back extensions	3 sets of 20	
Stretch		

DAYS 2, 4, AND 6 [WEEKS 19-21 CONTINUED]

Go for a 50-minute jog on all your cardio days during this three-week period.

WEEKS 22 - 24

DAYS 1, 3, AND 5

Exercise	Reps / Time / Weight	
Warm up/Stretch		
Treadmill	2 minutes high intensity	
Leg presses (feet low)	1 set of 10	75 lbs.
Leg extensions	1 set of 10	40 lbs.
Leg extensions	1 set of 10	20 lbs.
Leg presses (feet high)	1 set of 10	75 lbs.
Leg curls	1 set of 10	40 lbs.
Leg curls	1 set of 10	20 lbs.
Dumbbell chest presses	1 set of 10	12 lbs.
Dumbbell pec flies	1 set of 10	10 lbs.
Straight-bar cable pulldowns	1 set of 10	60 lbs.
Cable rows	1 set of 10	40 lbs.
Dumbbell chest presses	1 set of 10	12 lbs.
Dumbbell pec flies	1 set of 10	10 lbs.
Straight-bar cable pulldowns	1 set of 10	60 lbs.
Cable rows	1 set of 10	40 lbs.
Stationary bike	2 minutes high intensity	
Dumbbell squats	1 set of 10	12 lbs.
Step-ups	1 set of 10 per leg	12 lbs.
Plié squats	1 set of 10	12 lbs.
Stationary lunges	1 set of 10 per leg	12 lbs.
Dumbbell squats	1 set of 10	12 lbs.
Step-ups	1 set of 10 per leg	12 lbs.
Plie squats	1 set of 10	12 lbs.
Stationary lunges	1 set of 10 per leg	12 lbs.
Dumbbell shoulder presses	1 set of 10	12 lbs.
Lateral raises	1 set of 12	5 lbs.
Dumbbell bicep curls	1 set of 10	12 lbs.
Cable bicep curls	1 set of 12	25 lbs.
Tricep cable pushdowns	1 set of 10	40 lbs.
Bench dips	1 set of 12	
Dumbbell shoulder presses	1 set of 10	12 lbs.

DAYS 1, 3, AND 5 (WEEKS 22-24 CONTINUED)

Exercise	Reps / Time / Weight	
Lateral raises	1 set of 12	5 lbs.
Dumbbell bicep curls	1 set of 10	12 lbs.
Cable bicep curls	1 set of 12	25 lbs.
Tricep cable pushdowns	1 set of 10	40 lbs.
Bench dips	1 set of 12	
Hanging leg raises	1 set of 20	
Decline crunches	2 sets of 20	
Abs (on floor)	3 sets of 20	
Side bends	3 sets of 20 per side	
Lower back extensions	3 sets of 20	
Stretch		

DAYS 2, 4, AND 6

Go for a 48-minute interval jog on all your cardio days during this three-week period.

WEEKS 25-26

DAYS 1, 3, AND 5

Exercise	Reps / Time / Weight	
Warm up/Stretch		
Treadmill	30 sec. mod. intensity/30 sec. high intensity	
Leg extensions	1 set of 12	40 lbs.
Leg extensions	1 set of 12	20 lbs.
Leg curls	1 set of 12	40 lbs.
Leg curls	1 set of 12	20 lbs.
Leg presses (feet low)	1 set of 10	75 lbs.
Leg presses (feet high)	1 set of 10	75 lbs.
Dumbbell pec flies	1 set of 10	10 lbs.
Dumbbell chest presses	1 set of 10	12 lbs.
Cable rows	1 set of 10	40 lbs.
Straight-bar cable pulldowns	1 set of 10	60 lbs.
Dumbbell pec flies	1 set of 10	10 lbs.
Dumbbell chest presses	1 set of 10	12 lbs.
Cable rows	1 set of 10	40 lbs.
Straight-bar cable pulldowns	1 set of 10	60 lbs.
Stationary bike	30 sec. mod. intensity/30 sec. high intensity	
Step-ups	1 set of 10 per leg	12 lbs.
Dumbbell squats	1 set of 10	12 lbs.
Stationary lunges	1 set of 10 per leg	12 lbs.
Plie squats	1 set of 10	12 lbs.
Step-ups	1 set of 10 per leg	12 lbs.
Dumbbell squats	1 set of 10	12 lbs.
Stationary lunges	1 set of 10 per leg	12 lbs.
Plié squats	1 set of 10	12 lbs.
Lateral raises	1 set of 12	5 lbs.
Dumbbell shoulder presses	1 set of 10	12 lbs.
Cable bicep curls	1 set of 12	25 lbs.
Dumbbell bicep curls	1 set of 10	12 lbs.
Bench dips	1 set of 12	
Tricep cable pushdowns	1 set of 10	40 lbs.
Lateral raises	1 set of 12	5 lbs.
Dumbbell shoulder presses	1 set of 10	12 lbs.
Cable bicep curls	1 set of 12	25 lbs.
Dumbbell bicep curls	1 set of 10	12 lbs.
Bench dips	1 set of 12	
Tricep cable pushdowns	1 set of 10	40 lbs.

DAYS 1, 3, AND 5 (WEEKS 25-26 CONTINUED)

Exercise	Reps / Time / Weight
Hanging leg raises	2 sets of 20
Decline crunches	2 sets of 20
Abs (on floor)	2 sets of 20
Side bends	3 sets of 20 per side
Lower back extensions	3 sets of 20
Stretch	

DAYS 2, 4, AND 6

Go for a 50-minute jog on all your cardio days during these final two weeks.

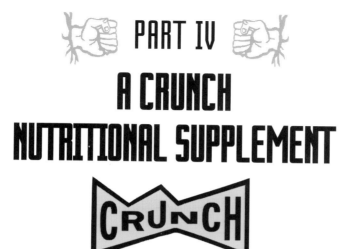

PART IV
A CRUNCH
NUTRITIONAL SUPPLEMENT

At CRUNCH, we believe in combining working out with eating right. Most people know that eating too much can sabotage their fitness efforts, but it is also crucial to eat the correct kinds of foods. Without the proper nutrients in the right ratios, you could be holding your body back from reaching its fitness potential. All it takes to get the most out of your workouts, to lose body fat, and to gain muscle is to educate yourself on the facts.

At CRUNCH Los Angeles, Eatwize™ Program directors Larry Krug and Brian Blacher with Jennifer Nardini, head of research and development, are using years' worth of testing, research, and real-world experience to bring clients the Eatwize™ Program, an individually tailored fat loss plan that really works. If you're looking to get as fit as you can as fast as you can, we can help you get the best results possible, safely. In order to take the guesswork out of the process, we've put together three different options tailored to accompany the workout you choose: four-week, three-month, and six-month programs of eating for maximum fat loss in minimum time. If you decide you like the way you look and feel after your designated time is up, we're also including a complete lifestyle program that you really can live with.

Before you begin, let's debunk a popular myth—that in order to lose weight, you need to exist on minute portions of food and feel completely miserable all the time. We Eatwize™ folks know that healthful eating isn't something to be dreaded or endured. Low-calorie, "crash" diets simply don't work. Period. Many clients come to us and swear that their friend lost weight on one of the high-protein, low-cal, high-carbohydrate, only fruit, no fruit, or any one of the myriad of diet trends out there today. The reality is that nearly all of the diets on the market at this time are just that—diets. They restrict calories to as low as 800 per day and offer the body up to all sorts of nutritional imbalances. This, coupled with the fact that any food plan that dips below 1,200 calories per day can cause your metabolism to slow down and hang on to your fat stores for dear life, makes most of these plans not only ineffective, but dangerous to your health.

Most weight lost on low-calorie diets, or any diet that causes you to lose more than two pounds a week, comes from water and muscle loss—not from fat. This is why so many people who claim to have lost weight on a crash diet regain it as soon as they have to start eating normally again. Plus, with less muscle and the same amount of fat, you won't be as toned or as energetic as you will be when you learn to eat more by eating "wize."

GENERAL GUIDELINES

Five principles are essential to the Eatwise™ Program's high success rate. They are as follows:

1. Aim for the 40-20-40 ratio. Optimally, you should combine your daily carbohydrate, fat, and protein into a 40-20-40 ratio. This does not mean that every food or every meal has to be a perfect 40-20-40 split, as long as your body maintains the 40-20-40 ratio in your system throughout the day.

It isn't enough to simply eat a 40-20-40 split of carbohydrates, fat, and protein. The Eatwise™ Program is about eating carbohydrates, proteins, and fats that are natural, low glycemic, and contain as few additives, preservatives, and chemicals as possible. The program also helps you get the right amount of vitamins, minerals, and antioxidants every day. The program allows you to enjoy your food while you lose weight. It is easy to follow and can adapt to your continually changing world by giving you the ability to make smart food choices anywhere you go.

We use this ratio as opposed to the more common 40-30-30 ratio because people who work out need more protein. Thirty percent fat simply ends up being too much for most people, especially since there are so many hidden fats in foods that even when you aim for 30% you may end up getting more.

2. Eat five small meals daily. To further optimize weight loss, we recommend eating three main meals and two snacks throughout the day. Any excess calories from an overload at any one meal may be stored as fat, so breaking it up can help ensure you don't exceed your threshold. Giving your body something to digest every three to four hours will leave you feeling satisfied as it keeps your metabolism working at a high level, thereby burning more fat.

Eating carbohydrates, which are sugars, causes your pancreas to release insulin, which transports sugar out of the blood, which in turn decreases your blood sugar levels. Eating protein releases glucagon, which transports sugars into the blood, causing your blood sugar levels to rise.

When you eat carbohydrates that cause your blood sugars to rise quickly, lots of insulin is released to deal with the overload. Too much insulin in your bloodstream can cause those carbohydrate sugars to be stored as fat.

Keeping your blood sugar levels stable seems to allow more of your fat stores to be accessed for fuel. To maintain steady blood sugar levels, combine complex carbohydrates, healthy fats, and lean proteins at each meal, or throughout the day in the best ratio we've found—40-20-40.

3. Eat fruits and vegetables. You've heard it before and you'll hear it again: Fruits are God's gift to healthful eaters. They're loaded with cancer-fighting vitamins and minerals. They deliver sugar in the form of fructose, which is more slowly absorbed into the body when wrapped in the high fiber of most whole fruits. Though they are a healthy way to satisfy your sweet tooth, certain fruits do cause a quick sugar release and are listed only on member profile C's food list (more on the food lists later). When following a fat-loss plan, it is best if you eat only one of these types of fruits a day, max.

Vegetables are God's other gift. Many health professionals are continuing to realize the powerful medicinal value of plants, touting them as the prevention or cure for most of our diseases. Above and beyond their excellent vitamin and mineral status, vegetables naturally contain phytochemicals, substances that protect them from their own diseases and outside toxins. Diets high in vegetables are also high in fiber, meaning that you can eat until you're full and still have many, many calories to spare. In addition, fiber keeps your colon cleansed, which is especially important to help prevent colon cancer and other intestinal problems.

4. Avoid saturated fat and refined and processed foods. So many people trying to lose weight are terrified of the fat gram. They've been taught that once any fat passes their lips, it immediately makes a beeline to join its many friends hanging out on their thighs and love handles. What many people don't know, however, is that eating fat is actually an important part of dropping pounds. Fat intake causes your body to let go of stored fat more easily. When you restrict your dietary fat substantially, your body thinks it needs to save what it already has in the event of a famine. So, follow the Eatwise™ guidelines and get 20 percent of your total daily calories from fat. Just make sure it's healthy fat like olive, avocado, canola, or peanut oils. Saturated fat, or fats derived from meat and other animal sources, like butter and cheese, are where other, healthier fats got their bad rap. Saturated fats contain cholesterol, as do some vegetable oils like palm and coconut oil. There seems to be little reason to eat saturated fat—it can clog your arteries, cause cancer, and is easily stored in your body.

Refined and over-processed foods can also present major stumbling blocks on your road to a strong, lean body. For starters, they can cause a big insulin release that may add to your fat stores. Since most of these foods (anything made with white flour or refined sugar, like cake, cookies, non-whole grain bagels, white bread—even rice cakes!) have little to no fiber content, they don't fill you up, and they are usually high in calories. Nor do they give you the sustained energy of their healthier, high-fiber counterparts, so you are likely to crash and crave even more of these carbs. Many people who think they are addicted to refined carbs, sugars, and fats are really caught in a vicious cycle of high and low blood sugar. To find out how to get off the roller coaster, read on!

5. Control your hormones. It is only human to fail on a restrictive, low-calorie diet. Your brain produces all sorts of chemicals to try to force you to eat if it thinks you are starving—and those chemicals are almost impossible to ignore. So what one person might call a failure, we at CRUNCH call heeding the call of survival. So this time, using the program, you will learn to circumvent your hormonal reactions by placating them with the right food combinations in the right amounts. Here are some of the most common reactions that occur in your body every time you eat.

Insulin. When you ingest carbohydrates, the hormone insulin is released by your pancreas into your bloodstream. Insulin's primary function is to transport blood sugar from the blood to your muscles and liver. Whenever insulin is released, carbohydrates become the body's primary source of energy. If you don't happen to be using much energy at the time, however, high levels of insulin may cause carbohydrates to be stored as fats.

Excess insulin in your system causes blood sugar levels to drop, which can result in disturbances in thinking, mood, or energy. When your blood sugar falls too low, it stimulates your appetite to eat more sugar, which produces more insulin. High insulin levels can thus wreak havoc on the system. When you get caught in the cycle, the only way you can get your sugar levels up again is to eat more sugar.

You can break the carbohydrate cycle by eating the right amount of fat and protein in your daily diet and the right amount of unrefined or low-glycemic carbohydrates. With the correct combinations, you can regulate the body's insulin levels and reduce your previously out-of-control cravings.

Glucagon. The pancreas releases glucagon into the bloodstream as part of the digestive process. Glucagon has the opposite effect from insulin. It releases sugar from the muscle and liver back into the bloodstream. This helps to maintain and stabilize blood sugar levels and allows the body to release fat for energy.

Glucagon releases carbohydrates into the bloodstream to be broken down into calories. Glucagon is stimulated by protein, therefore it is important to eat protein with carbohydrates to keep insulin and glucagon levels in balance. This is one reason the 40-20-40 ratio works so well.

The glycemic index. The glycemic index is a scale that rates how fast food becomes glucose in your bloodstream and therefore how much insulin is secreted to help metabolize that food. If a food has a low glycemic index, less insulin is released and the amount of glucose derived from that food is sustained in the bloodstream over a longer period of time. This is a good thing, because stable blood sugar means less fat stored and more released.

Food with a high glycemic index causes the release of more insulin more rapidly. The glucose will last for a shorter period of time, which in turn may cause you to become hungry more quickly, and you'll run out of energy faster.

Lucky for you, we've removed the guesswork for you. The foods on the member profile A list (see page 124) are generally low glycemic, those for member B are mostly medium glycemic, and those for member C are generally high glycemic. In order to maximize weight loss,

THE EATWISE™ PRINCIPLES FOR EATING OUT

- Avoid eating the bread when it is brought to the table.
- Have a small snack before going to a restaurant in case it takes a while before you get your food.
- Consider splitting your meal with somebody—many restaurants serve very large portions.
- Order salads with dressing on the side.
- Do not order cream-based foods.
- Tell the server exactly how you want your food prepared.
- Always share your dessert if you decide to order one.
- Asked for steamed veggies, not sautéed.
- Save your member C foods for when you eat out, when you always have less control.

always aim for the low glycemic foods. (Note: We have rated our food choices by other factors, such as how natural it is, and how many sugars, additives, and preservatives it contains. Not all foods for member A are completely low glycemic, but they may have other redeeming properties that make them perfectly acceptable choices).

HOW TO MAKE SENSE OF FOOD LABELS

Here's more guesswork out the window, courtesy of Eatwize™. When beginning a new eating plan, it's smart to stock your personal space at home or work with healthful foods you can easily prepare. Here's a breakdown on how to read a standard food label, as well as a breakdown of the terminology.

Consider this example of a label of 2% low-fat milk:

Nutrition Facts

Serving size	1 cup (240ml)
Servings per container	about 2

Percent daily values are based on a 2,000 calorie diet. Your daily values may be higher or lower based on your caloric needs.

	Amount per serving	% daily value
Calories	130	
Calories from fat	45	
Total fat	5 g	8 %
Saturated fat	3 g	5 %
Cholesterol	2 mg	8 %
Sodium	130 mg	5 %
Total Carbohydrates	13 g	4 %
Dietary fiber	0 g	0 %
Sugars	13 g	
Protein	10 g	19 %
Vitamin A		10 %
Vitamin C		4 %
Calcium		35 %
Iron		0 %
Vitamin D		25 %

The above figures are based on the caloric needs of a person on a 2,000 calorie-a-day diet. Here are the needs of a 2,500 calorie-a-day diet, for comparison:

Calories	2,000	2,500
Total fat	less than 6 g	80 g
Saturated fat	less than 20 g	25 g
Cholesterol	less than 30 mg	300 mg
Sodium	less than 2,400 mg	2,400 mg
Total Carbohydrates	less than 300 g	375 g
Dietary Fiber	25 g	30 g
Protein	50 g	65 g

1. Look at the serving size (1 cup).
2. Check to see how many servings are in the container (2 servings).
3. See how many calories are in the serving (130 calories).
4. Look how many calories are from fat (45 calories).
5. Determine the percentage of total calories coming from fat. The maximum calories from fat should not exceed 20%. Calories from fat divided by total calories per serving is equal to the percentage of calories coming from fat. If this percentage is more than 20% there is too much fat (45 divided by 130 = 32%).
6. Don't be fooled by the percentages given in the right hand column. Those numbers refer to the Recommended Daily Allowances. For example, in 2% fat milk, the calories from fat are not

2% of the total calories, but 32%. Check to see how much fat and what type of fat is in the product.

7. See how much sugar is in the product. On this label, all 13 grams of carbohydrates are pure sugar.

Fat-free labels are usually high in sugar and chemicals, and unfortunately, fat-free does not mean calorie-free. Sugar is often substituted for taste instead of fat.

Did you know that a food can be labeled calorie-free and still have calories? According to the American Heart Association, the following criteria must be met when making certain claims about food:

- Calorie-Free: fewer than 5 calories.
- Light (Lite): One-third fewer calories, or no more than half the fat or sodium of the regular versions.
- Fat-Free: less than 0.5 gram of fat.
- Low Fat: no more than 3 grams of fat.
- Reduced or Less Fat: at least 25% less fat.
- Lean: less than 10 grams of fat, 4 grams of saturated fat, and 95 mg of cholesterol.
- Extra Lean: less than 5 grams of fat, 2 grams, and 95 mg. of cholesterol.
- Low in Saturated Fat: no more than 1 gram of fat and 15% of calories from saturated fat.
- Cholesterol Free: less than 2 mg. cholesterol and 2 grams of saturated fat.
- Low Cholesterol: no more than 20 mg. of cholesterol and 2 grams of saturated fat.
- Reduced Cholesterol: at least 25% less cholesterol and 2 grams or less of saturated fat.
- Sodium Free: fewer than 5 mg. of sodium and no sodium chloride.
- Very Low Sodium: 35 or fewer mg. of sodium.
- Low Sodium: no more than 140 mg. of sodium.
- Reduced or Less Sodium: at least 25% less sodium.
- Sugar Free: less than 0.5 gram of sugar.
- No added sugar: means no added sucrose—however, it could mean that the food is sweetened with honey, syrups, or fruit juice.
- Low Sugar: Less than 5% of total weight.
- Unsweetened fruit juice may have no added sugar, but fruit juice *is* sugar.
- Sugar free, fat free, dairy free: If the product is sugar free, fat free, dairy free, taste free etc., it does not mean it is calorie free—it will still have carbohydrates or protein.

- High Fiber: at least 5 grams of fiber.
- Good Source of Fiber: 2.5 to 4.9 grams of fiber.

WHICH MEMBER PROFILE DO YOU FIT?

Here at CRUNCH L.A., our trainers and nutritionists often deal with actors and actresses who need to whip themselves into shape quickly for a movie or a photo shoot. Of course, so-called "real people" have their own emergency situations to deal with as well. Say you promised to be a bridesmaid in your friend's wedding and six months ago, when they fit you for the dress, you were sure that you'd be one size smaller than you are right now. You've got a month to get it together and you need a plan that works. For those with limited time before an important event, try our four-week program. This is the safest way to lose the most weight in a short period of time. Eat less, and you risk lowering your metabolism and storing fat. The same goes if you try to continue on with the four-week program for longer than the allotted time. But for a smart quick fix, this plan can't be beat.

On the first day of the four-week program, write down your starting weight and body fat percentage. You can have a personal trainer or a nutritionist test your body fat, or go to your local gym if you're unfamiliar with the process. Then, record your new, improved stats once a week. The average client can expect to lose roughly two pounds a week, about eight to ten pounds total. That works out to be a 4% loss. While this may not sound like a lot, you'll be losing pure fat and gaining muscle, so the results will really show.

After the four weeks are up, if you want to keep up your progress, move on to the three-month plan so you don't experience a rebound effect and regain any weight.

If you have a little longer to prepare until you need to be leaner, try our three-month program. It offers a bit more leeway when it comes to food choices and the calorie levels are slightly increased. These two factors make the three-month period more manageable for the average person. You'll have more to work with, and with 12 weeks to go, you should have no problem losing a substantial amount of fat.

We predict that in three months, you'll be able to lose between 10 to 15 pounds, or 4 to 8% body fat.

We'll back off even more if we know you've got six whole months to transform yourself. You'll get even more calories and you can even eat one not-so-good-for-you-but-oh-so-good food every day from each category. The six-month plan enables you to fully integrate the Eatwise™ principles into a lifestyle change, and if you so desire, you may continue the plan past the six-month cutoff and make healthy eating a permanent part of your everyday life. With such an ample amount of time, you can expect to lose anywhere from five to 25 pounds of fat, or 10 to 15% total.

Of course, the amount you lose on any of these plans may vary from what other people experience, based on your current body composition, activity level, and genetic factors. Obviously, the more closely you stick to the plan, the better your results will be.

FREE VEGETABLES

No matter which plan you choose, feel free to have as many of these veggies as you like without counting them toward your daily calorie totals.

Arame	Collard Greens	Peppers
Artichokes	Cucumber	Radishes
Arugula	Dulse	Rhubarb
Asparagus	Eggplant	Rutabaga
Bamboo Shoots	Endives	Scallions
Beetroot	Green Beans	Spinach
Bok Choy	Jicama	Sprouts
Broccoli	Kale	Swiss Chard
Cabbage	Kelp	Tomatoes
Cauliflower	Lettuce	Turnips
Celery	Kohlrabi	Water Chestnuts
Chicory	Mushroom	Watercress
Chives	Onions	Zucchini

FREE FOODS

These are foods you can also have in moderation without counting them as part of your daily intake:

Condiments
Anchovelle Paste
Ketchup
Garlic
Horseradish
Lemon Juice
Mint
Ginger
Mustard
Salsa
Soy Sauce (light)
Spices
Tamarind
Tobasco
Vinegar
Wasabi

Drinks
Coffee*
Tea*
Herbal Tea
Wheatgrass Juice
Diet Soda*
Non Caloric Drinks

Foods
Diet Jell-O
Non-Calorie Foods
Cucumbers (pickled)

*Not more than one cup a day

MEMBER PROFILE A: THE FOUR-WEEK PLAN

	Women	**Men**
Calories:	1,200 to 1,400	1,400 to 1,800
Carbohydrates:	4 to 5 medium-size	6 to 7 servings per
day		
	servings per day.	
	(approx. 100 calories)	
Fats:	2 servings per day	3 servings per day
Protein:	4 to 5 servings per day	5 to 6 servings daily

Carbohydrate List:

A small serving (3 oz.) of:

Apple, Apricots, Barley, Berries, Cereal (high fiber, no sugar), Cherries, Grapefruit, Guava, Lentils, Oatmeal, Peas, Plums, Pumpkin, Rice (brown, basmati), Squash, Strawberries, Sweet Potatoes, Tangerine, Vegetable Garden Burger

These carbs have the lowest glycemic rating, the lowest amounts of sugar and are the least refined and processed.

Fat List

A small serving (3 oz.) of:

20% of your daily intake can come from the following unsaturated fats: Avocado, Nuts (all), Oils (olive, canola, flaxseed sesame, soybean), Olives, Pumpkin Seeds

Protein List:

A small serving (3 oz.) of:

Chicken Breast, Egg, Egg Whites, Fish (white fish), Protein Powders (all), Soya Burger (fat free), Tofu (low fat, low sodium), Tuna (canned, white, in water), Turkey Breast (white meat)

These proteins are the highest quality of protein with the least amount of saturated bad fats.

MEMBER PROFILE B: THE THREE-MONTH PLAN

	Women	Men
Calories:	1,200 to 1,400	1,400 to 1,800
Carbohydrates: day	4 to 5 medium-size	6 to 7 servings per
	servings per day. (approx. 100 calories)	
Fats:	2 servings per day	3 servings per day
Protein:	4 to 5 servings per day	5 to 6 servings daily

Member B can include the following foods in addition to all the foods on subject A's list. When choosing your carbohydrates from the following list, women should not exceed 5 medium-sized (approximately 100 calories) of these servings per day.

Carbohydrate List:

A small serving (3 oz.) of:

Bananas, Bread (high fiber, low sugar), Buckwheat, Bulgar Wheat, Cereal (high-fiber, low-sugar), Corn, Cous-Cous, Fruit Salad (citrus, no sugar), Fruit Snacks (dried, no sugar), Grapes, Grits, Honey, Kiwi, Nectarine, Noodles (soba and udon), Oat Bran (hot cereal).

Fat List:

A small serving (3 oz.) of:

Coconut, Guacamole, Humus, Oil (corn, peanut, sunflower), Nut Butters (almond, cashew, etc.), Peanut Butter (light, natural), Salad Dressing (low fat, no cream), Sesame Seeds, Sunflower Seeds.

Protein List:

A small serving (3 oz.) of:

Cottage Cheese (low fat), Cottage Cheese (fat free), Fish (pink), Hot Dog (tofu, fat-free), Vegetarian Protein Burger, Ground Turkey (97% lean), Scallops, Shrimp, Prawns, Oysters, Turkey Slice (fat free).

MEMBER PROFILE C: THE SIX-MONTH PLAN

	Women	Men
Calories:	1,200 to 1,400	1,400 to 1,800
Carbohydrates:	4 to 5 medium-size	6 to 7 servings per day
	servings per day. (approx. 100 calories)	
Fats:	2 servings per day	3 servings per day
Protein:	4 to 5 servings per day	5 to 6 serving daily

Member C can choose from any of the carbs recommended for Members A and B. However, Member C can add one serving per day of the following foods. Member C women can have 5 to 7 servings per day of carbs, and men can have 7 to 9 servings per day.

Carbohydrate List (do not exceed 1 serving a day from this list):

Applesauce (non-sugar), Bagel, Baguette, Beer (light or regular), White Bread/Roll/Pita, Canned Fruit (non-sugar) , Cantaloupe, Carrot Juice, Carrots, Cereal (low sugar), Chips (low fat), Cornstarch, Crackers (salty), Crackers/Cookies (sweet), Cream of Wheat, Croissant/Muffin, Croutons, Dried Fruit (mixed), Figs, Flour (all), Frozen Yogurt (nonfat), Fruit Juice (all).

Fat List (do not exceed 1 serving a day from this list):

Butter, Dips (cream-based), Margarine, Marinades, BBQ Sauces, Mayonnaise (light), Palm Oil, Pesto Sauce, Salad Dressing (low fat, cream)

Protein List (do not exceed 1 serving a day from this list):

Beef (93% lean ground), Beef Burger, Beef Steak (lean), Sirloin Fillet, Cold Cut (lean), Duck, Lamb, Pork

Keep track of your progress with the following chart:

Week	Date	Weight (lbs.)	Body fat %	Fat loss in %	Weight loss (in lbs.)
1					
2					

IT'S JUST A NUMBER

You really can't tell much from staring at the numbers on the scale. They can't tell you how much of your total weight comes from fat, muscle, bone, or water. Only a professional fat percentage or body composition test can tell you that. It is possible to lose fat, gain muscle, drop a dress size, feel and look great, and still gain weight! Muscle weighs more per area than fat does, so make certain that you look to your body fat testing for the real scoop on your progress. To help you decode the numbers you'll get back, here is a chart of body-fat ranges.

MALES (% BODY FAT)

Age	Excellent	Very Good	Good	Average	Fair	Poor
19–24	6–10	11–13	14–17	18–21	22–25	> 25
25–29	6–10	11–14	15–18	19–22	23–26	> 26
30–34	6–10	11–15	16–19	20–23	24–27	> 27
35–39	6–10	11–16	17–20	21–24	25–28	> 28
40–44	6–10	11–17	18–21	22–25	26–29	> 29
45–49	6–10	11–18	19–22	23–26	27–30	> 30
50+	6–10	11–19	20–23	24–27	28–31	> 31

FEMALES (% BODY FAT)

Age	Excellent	Very Good	Good	Average	Fair	Poor
18–24	8–12	13–15	16–19	20–23	24–27	> 27
25–29	8–12	13–16	17–20	21–24	25–28	> 28
30–34	8–12	13–17	18–21	22–25	26–29	> 29
35–39	8–12	13–18	19–22	23–26	27–30	> 30
40–44	8–12	13–19	20–23	24–27	28–31	> 31
45–49	8–12	13–20	21–24	25–28	29–32	> 32
50+	8–12	13–21	22–25	26–29	30–33	> 33

MAINTENANCE

It's certainly possible and definitely exciting to get fit in a crunch. Once you see how much difference finding an eating program that compliments your workouts can make, you'll probably want to make it a permanent addition to your life. If you began on program A, move to program B, then on to program C. If you started program B, move to program C after the three months are up. Once on program C, you can feel comfortable continuing indefinitely.

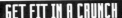

Please consult your physician before starting any nutritional program. This is only part of the Eatwize™ Program—log onto **www.eatwize.com** for more information.

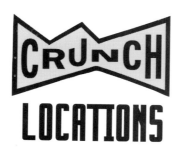

LOCATIONS

Where to work out, pretend to work out, or just stand around calling our personal trainers "Hans" and "Franz" under your breath.

NEW YORK CITY

404 Lafayette Street
(Astor Place and 4th Avenue)
212.614.0120

54 East 13th Street
(University and Broadway)
212.475.2018

162 West 83rd Street
(Columbus and Amsterdam)
212.875.1902

623 Broadway (at Houston)
212.420.0507

152 Christopher Street
(at Greenwich Street)
212.366.3725

1109 Second Avenue
(at 59th Street)
212.758.3434

144 W. 38th St.
(7th Ave. & Broadway)
212.869.7788

LOS ANGELES

8000 Sunset Blvd.
(West Hollywood)
323.654.4550

MISSION VIEJO

The Kaleidoscope Center
27741 Crown Valley Parkway
949.582.8181

SAN FRANCISCO

1000 Van Ness Avenue
(Geary and O'Farrell)
415.931.1100

MIAMI

1259 Washington Avenue
(South Beach)
305.674.8222

ATLANTA AREA
[ALL LOCATIONS: 800.660.5433]

Crunch Club Cobb
North by NW Office Park
1775 Water Place
Atlanta, GA 30339

Crunch Gwinnett
Gwinnett Prado
2300 Pleasant Hill Road
Duluth, GA 30136

Crunch Town Center
Main Street Shopping Center
2600 Prado Lane
Marietta, GA 30066

Crunch Roswell
Roswell Exchange
11060 Alpharetta Highway
Roswell, GA 30076

Crunch Buckhead
3365 Piedmont Road, Suite 1010
Atlanta, GA

Crunch Stone Mountain
Stone Mountain Square
5370 Highway 78 South
Stone Mountain, GA 30087

TOKYO

Crunch Omotesando
4-3-24 Jingumae Sibuya

Coming soon to Las Vegas and Chicago!

Visit us on the Web at
www.crunch.com

Have questions about this workout?

Ask the authors at:

WWW.GETFITNOW.COM

*The **hottest** fitness spot on the internet!*

FEATURING . . .

"Ask the Expert" Q&A Boards

Stimulating Discussion groups

Cool Links

Great Photos

Full-Motion Videos

Downloads

The Five Star Fitness Team

Hot Product Reviews

And More!

Log on today to receive a FREE catalog

or call us at

1-800-906-1234

Fit Test / Personal Training Session

15% OFF! 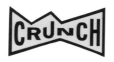 15% OFF!

IT'S EASY . . . Come into any CRUNCH location and receive 15% off your first purchase of personal training. Then just sign, date, and present this coupon at the fitness desk to set up your session.

_____   _____
MEMBER NAME   SIGNATURE

_____   _____
TRAINER NAME   TRAINER SIGNATURE

_____
DATE OF SESSION

Cannot be combined with any other offer. Valid for one use only

---- CUT AT DOTTED LINE ----

GUEST PASS

$22 value!
Must show picture ID to use facility.
The same guest may use only two guest passes per year

_____   _____
MEMBERSHIP REP   EXPIRATION DATE

OUR MISSION AND PHILOSOPHY

We at CRUNCH warmly welcome people from all walks of life,
regardless of shape, size, sex, or ability.
People don't have to be flawless to feel at home at CRUNCH. We don't care
if our members are 18 or 80, fat or thin, short or tall, muscular or mushy, blond or bald,
or anywhere in between. CRUNCH is not competitive, it is non-judgmental,
it is not elitist, it does not represent a kind of person.
CRUNCH is a gym; a movement which is growing as we continue to perfect our ability
to create an environment where our members don't feel self-conscious,
and don't worry about what others think.
At the heart of CRUNCH's core stands a tremendously experienced and energetic staff
dedicated to creating an environment where everyone feels accepted—
a truly unique place!

WWW.CRUNCH.COM

The **hottest** fitness spot on the internet!

OUR MISSION AND PHILOSOPHY

We at CRUNCH warmly welcome people from all walks of life,
regardless of shape, size, sex, or ability.
People don't have to be flawless to feel at home at CRUNCH. We don't care
if our members are 18 or 80, fat or thin, short or tall, muscular or mushy, blond or bald,
or anywhere in between. CRUNCH is not competitive, it is non-judgmental,
it is not elitist, it does not represent a kind of person.
CRUNCH is a gym; a movement which is growing as we continue to perfect our ability
to create an environment where our members don't feel self-conscious,
and don't worry about what others think.
At the heart of CRUNCH's core stands a tremendously experienced and energetic staff
dedicated to creating an environment where everyone feels accepted—
a truly unique place!

WWW.CRUNCH.COM

*The **hottest** fitness spot on the internet!*

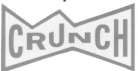

- - - CUT AT DOTTED LINE - - -

NEW YORK CITY

404 Lafayette Street
(Astor Place and 4th Street)
212.614.0120

54 East 13th Street
(University and Broadway)
212.475.2018

162 West 83rd Street
(Columbus and Amsterdam)
212.875.1902

623 Broadway (at Houston)
212.420.0507

152 Christopher Street
(at Greenwich Street)
212.366.3725

1109 Second Avenue
(at 59th Street)
212.758.3434

144 W. 38th St.
(7th Ave. & Broadway)
212.869.7788

LOS ANGELES

8000 Sunset Blvd.
(West Hollywood)
323.654.4550

SAN FRANCISCO

1000 Van Ness Avenue
(Geary and O'Farrell)
415.931.1100

MISSION VIEJO

The Kaleidoscope Center
27741 Crown Valley
    Parkway
949.582.8181

MIAMI

1259 Washington Avenue
(South Beach)
305.674.8222

ATLANTA AREA
(All locations: 800.660.5433)

Crunch Club Cobb
North by NW Office Park
1775 Water Place
Atlanta, GA 30339

Crunch Gwinnett
Gwinnett Prado
2300 Pleasant Hill Road
Duluth, GA 30136

Crunch Town Center
Main Street Shopping
    Center
2600 Prado Lane
Marietta, GA 30066

Crunch Roswell
Roswell Exchange
11060 Alpharetta Highway
Roswell, GA 30076

Crunch Buckhead
3365 Piedmont Road,
Suite 1010
Atlanta, GA

Crunch Stone Mountain
Stone Mountain Square
5370 Highway 78 South
Stone Mountain, GA 30087

TOKYO

Crunch Omotesando
4-3-24 Jingumae Sibuya

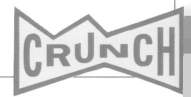

CHICAGO AND LAS VEGAS COMING SOON!